AN OPEN AND SHUT CASE

The Story of Keyhole or Minimally Invasive Surgery

AN OPEN AND SHUT CASE

The Story of Keyhole or Minimally Invasive Surgery

John Wickham

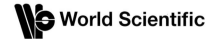

World Scientific

NEW JERSEY · LONDON · SINGAPORE · BEIJING · SHANGHAI · HONG KONG · TAIPEI · CHENNAI · TOKYO

Published by

World Scientific Publishing Europe Ltd.

57 Shelton Street, Covent Garden, London WC2H 9HE

Head office: 5 Toh Tuck Link, Singapore 596224

USA office: 27 Warren Street, Suite 401-402, Hackensack, NJ 07601

Library of Congress Cataloging-in-Publication Data
Names: Wickham, J. E. A. (John Ewart Alfred), author.
Title: An open and shut case : the story of keyhole or minimally invasive surgery /
    by John Wickham.
Description: New Jersey : World Scientific, 2017.
Identifiers: LCCN 2016045894| ISBN 9781786341716 (hc : alk. paper) |
    ISBN 9781786341723 (pbk : alk. paper)
Subjects: | MESH: Wickham, J. E. A. (John Ewart Alfred) | Minimally Invasive
    Surgical Procedures--history | Robotic Surgical Procedures--history | Urologic Surgical
    Procedures--history | History, 20th Century | Great Britain | Autobiography
Classification: LCC RD33.53 | NLM WZ 100 | DDC 617/.05--dc23
LC record available at https://lccn.loc.gov/2016045894

British Library Cataloguing-in-Publication Data
A catalogue record for this book is available from the British Library.

Desk Editors: V. Vishnu Mohan/Mary Simpson

Typeset by Stallion Press
Email: enquiries@stallionpress.com

Printed in Singapore by Mainland Press Pte Ltd.

*"It is surely a gross presumption to dismantle
the image of God"*

John Woodall

Barber Surgeon 1556–1643

Worshipful Company of Barber Surgeons, London

About the Author

Mr J. E. A. Wickham BSc (Hon), MB, BS, MD (Hon), FRCS (Eng), FRCP (Hon), FRCR (Hon), FRSM (Hon) was Senior Urological Surgeon and Head of the Department of Urology, St Bartholomew's Hospital London. He was Director of the Academic Unit at the Institute of Urology, University of London at St Peter's Postgraduate Urological Hospitals and at the Middlesex Hospital London. He was Consultant Urological Surgeon at Ring Edward VII Hospital London and served as Civilian Consultant in Urology to The Royal Air Force. He was also Honorary Research Lecturer and Consultant Surgeon, Guy's Hospital London.

Foreword

I first met John Wickham in 2011, when I started researching the early days of keyhole surgery. I realised that there were very few first-hand accounts of what actually happened during those remarkable decades which turned traditional surgery on its head. Since then I have interviewed John on many occasions, filmed him and his colleagues performing simulated re-enactments of early keyhole surgery, and got to know him as a man. Over the years that followed I became fascinated with John's story and the pivotal yet under-recognised part he played.

The second half of John's book — his personal account of the early days of what became keyhole surgery — gives a fascinating insight into that surgical world. It chronicles how John and his colleagues broke new ground in urinary tract stone surgery, how they carried out the first percutaneous nephrolithotomy, how they pioneered extracorporeal shockwave lithotripsy in the UK and how they developed the first autonomous surgical robot. But these were only prominent moments in a lifelong career of innovation and invention, driven by a determination to minimise the damage done by traditional open surgery and improve the experience of patients.

These events are given a rich background by the book's first section. John's account of what it was like to be a medical student and trainee surgeon in the 1950s and 1960s opens a door onto a vanished world. Though vestiges of that world were still in place when I was a medical student and a surgical trainee, it now seems unimaginably distant. Yet, understanding that context is essential to making sense of John's later contributions.

Alongside these accounts of pivotal developments in the world of surgery runs an unfolding sense of John Wickham the man. His life outside surgery — his family, his passion for restoring old sports cars, his relentless drive to fix mechanical things — captures his restless energy. His personal qualities — his ability to inspire others, to establish and lead a team of innovators at the Institute of Urology, to develop a revolutionary vision of minimally invasive therapy — are striking. Yet, this emerges gradually from John's writing style, with its wry humour, self-deprecating stories and his gentle (and sometimes not so gentle) irony. His book gives the sense of a reformer and a constant innovator who inspires and supports his colleagues — but also of someone who has no time for incompetence or laziness, who does not suffer fools gladly or put up with those who do not share his commitment to patient care. Uncompromisingly honest about his own failures, he mercilessly dissects the reasons why some of his ventures did not succeed.

It would be easy to focus on a list of John's individual achievements and see him as a technical innovator, a pioneer of surgical techniques. Of course, he was that. But his contribution runs far deeper. A contrarian and a visionary thinker, he has continually reached beyond his own practice to ask bigger questions, to challenge and provoke. His ideal of minimally invasive therapy as a principle applicable across surgery, not just within urology, is now widely accepted. But it is easy to forget how radical a vision this was at the time, and how much opprobrium he had to endure.

John's refusal to be confined by the status quo has helped to shape some of the most convulsive changes in twentieth century surgery. Controversial, challenging and revolutionary in his thinking yet gentle, courteous and urbane as a man, John Wickham is one of the major surgical figures of his time. This fascinating account of his life, his achievements and his thinking fills a major gap for surgeons, historians and the general reader. It could not have come at a better time.

Roger Kneebone
Professor of Surgical Education
and Engagement Science
Imperial College London

Acknowledgements

So many persons have influenced the decisions recorded in this narrative that any individual recognition is difficult.

Consideration in groups therefore seems sensible.

Firstly, mentors. My clinical teachers were vastly important in progressing my career especially John O'Connell, Alec Badenoch, Ronald Bodley-Scott, Peter Martin, and Ben Eiseman. Without their practical and wise guidance I could not have succeeded in what I did.

Secondly, my junior medical colleagues. These were vitally helpful in the realisation of a number of projects I pursued over 30 years. I would single out Michael Kellett, Ron Miller, John Fitzpatrick, Malcom Coptcoat, John Ward, David Webb, and Brian Davies all mentioned in the text.

Associated with this group who were not physicians were the many specialists in their own disciplines. Other ancillary helpers were the physicists, photographers, computer experts, and especially the Instrument makers like Stuart Greengrass of Olympus Ltd.

The influence of various secretaries over all these years has been immense. All have been amazingly competent and loyal from Erica Shapiro at the start of my practice followed by Lindsey Frost and to the star final performer Anneka Wright who has laboured away so expertly over a 20-year period and recently interpreted my hideous writing into legible type script for this small presentation.

The staff of World Scientific, Merlin Fox, Mary Simpson and Vishnu Mohan have guided me in the mysteries of publishing and I am very grateful.

Professor Roger Kneebone stimulated me to get out of my armchair and suggested I should record some of my experiences in a practice of Surgery over a 30-year period. I hope he was wise?

Now my family — my wife and three daughters now with seven grandchildren and Boris — whose IT and other knowledge have contributed in various ways I would also like to thank.

Finally, I would like to thank my wife for many years of encouragement, and practical help in so many ways which enabled me to follow this somewhat tortuous and demanding Career path. To Her, I should like to dedicate this small volume with all my love and gratitude for all her care and tolerance of a rather strange human organism!

Contents

PART II — The Adventures of the Fully Trained Surgeon! 117

PART I

How, Why, What?

Since retiring, I have been asked on several occasions three questions:

Firstly, why did you become a surgeon? The short answer is — Not by any deliberate plan, but by following a path that spontaneously appeared in front of me.

Secondly, how did you become a surgeon? The short answer — With a little difficulty and effort.

Thirdly, what was it like to be a surgeon? The short answer — The most truly satisfying combination of a practical and intellectual activity that I can conceive and that I had the privilege to participate in.

The long answers deserve a degree of expansion and require a personal biographical record which at times may be boring, but hopefully may be interesting. The reader must be the judge.

The period that I record refers to the four decades when I worked in Medicine and Surgery in various capacities from 1950 to the 1990s.

Much has been written of the developments in surgery arising from military experiences during the two world wars of 1914–1918 and 1939–1945, but I refer to events that I experienced in United Kingdom civilian practice.

This period coincides with the establishment of the United Kingdom National Health Service and the changes in medical and nursing practice that this induced.

Chapter 1

School and War

Firstly, let me share my earlier background and how I was steered into a medical career.

No one in my family had been medically qualified although several had been in the nursing profession. I was born in 1927 in Chichester, West Sussex to a middle class family. My father was involved in what would now be called Event Management, namely the organisation of social events such as wedding parties, garden parties, racing parties, balls and other similar events. The business was based in West Sussex in Chichester, and had other branches in Bognor Regis, and Littlehampton while my grandfather conducted the other part of the organisation in Surrey with facilities based in Weybridge, Reigate and Dorking.

It was a complete disaster in 1931–1933 when both my grandfather and father died within 18 months of each other bringing the whole organisation to a sudden halt. When all was sorted out, there was a small income for grandmother and mother which just managed to achieve financial stability.

After my father died at the age of 42 from pneumonia and pulmonary embolism, I lived with my widowed mother in a flat on the seafront in Littlehampton in Sussex (see Fig. 1.1) from 1937 until we moved away from the seafront in 1941 because of coastal bombing and other military events. For instance, two large naval guns were mounted on the promenade directly opposite to our flat which

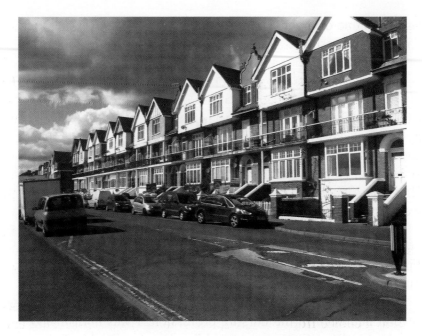

Fig. 1.1. South Terrace, Littlehampton, Sussex.

on the two occasions they were fired acoustically shattered a number of windows on the seafront houses. A second event which galvanised my mother and thrilled me was the sight from our front window of a Messerschmitt Bf109 followed closely by two Hurricanes at about 200 ft which had to pull up to avoid buildings at the end of the harbour! Few memories remain of these years, but a feeling of sadness seemed to pervade the family home. One other complicating factor comes to mind. I apparently developed ringworm of the scalp from putting on the school cap of a child suffering from the disease. My poor mother became frantic as all the medication appeared useless. An aunt who was a Sister at the London Hospital consulted a Dermatologist who recommended a course of epilation radiotherapy. My mother had to sign a declaration that if no hair grew again, the hospital would not be responsible. I had the deep X-ray treatment and I was cured and happily my hair grew again until my early twenties when it gradually disappeared again. As one of my chiefs remarked being bald would put another £50 on any consultation in Harley Street! This was much later.

I had attended a rather indifferent local preparatory school aged 8–9 and any thought of public school to follow was not possible. To my surprise, I managed to pass the entrance examination to Chichester High School for Boys in 1939, a Grammar school set up by the Sussex County Authorities in 1922. The staff were excellent and all had university degrees. I think we had a good education with at least half of our sixth form of 30 or so pupils proceeding to University, quite unusual at that time and, of that number, seven went to Oxford or Cambridge.

As an average student, I passed my Oxford School Certificate in 1944 with credits in English Language, English Literature, Mathematics, Physics, Chemistry and Biology with enough grades to advance into the sixth form.

I had been more interested in Science than Arts and I was offered a choice from two groups of four subjects: either Pure and Applied Mathematics plus Physics and Chemistry or Botany, Zoology, Physics and Chemistry. As my mathematical abilities were limited, I opted for the latter four subjects and was unknowingly steered towards medicine as a career.

World War Two was proceeding noisily during most of my time at school and living on the south coast in Sussex provided quite a few, if not dangerously exciting moments. My daily journey to school by train pulled by an old-fashioned steam tank engine was in its own right quite an adventure. I left home at 8.00 am and caught the train at 8.15 am for the slow journey to Chichester. Along the route, we picked up other boys attending the school from Bognor Regis and surrounding villages. En route there was plenty of opportunity for sport such as placing smaller boys in the luggage racks, unscrewing and removing the rather nice adverts for seaside summer holidays on the 'Sussex Riviera' from the carriage walls, and dodging the train guard which was not difficult as all the carriages were of the old eight seater compartment type with no corridor access.

On the return journey, there was often much activity from war-ring aircraft overhead and one afternoon our train was 'shot up' by a Focke Wolf 190. There was a bit of broken glass, but no one was seriously injured apart from the engine which was disabled and was sprouting steam from various unnatural orifices. As boys we thoroughly enjoyed the experience arriving home four hours late to be met by groups of anxious mothers. While we were thrilled. 'Mum we've been shot up', etc. The mothers, white with anxiety, were less impressed.

Another memory was of prisoners of war, usually Italians, being paraded in Chichester station car park at our arrival time, prior to being taken out to local farms to work. On the day Mussolini was reported to have been killed, one of my school friends stood in front of these men saying as he drew his hand, across his throat 'Mussolini Dead'. Whereupon one of the Italians jumped forward and seized him by the throat and he was nearly strangled before the guards pulled him off. Just like a movie!

At school, our lessons were frequently interrupted by air raid warnings when we had to proceed to windowless, unilluminated brick built structures in the school playing fields. It was impossible to conduct any meaningful instruction here and quite a few hours were given up in joking about in the dark. Some of the masters read us improving literature by torch light, others read adventure stories such as John Buchan which concentrated our attention.

Outside things were much more interesting with dog-fights going on overhead, the odd plane falling from the sky and crashing nearby. Collecting pieces of crashed aircraft or other armaments was a common form of currency. 'I'll swap you a bit of Heinkel III for a piece of Spitfire', etc. One could pick up spent cannon shell cases and the solid cannon shells themselves which had been fired by the fighters overhead and which had fallen all around in the street avoiding the potentially explosive ones! I still have one in front of me now. Another sport was to collect the unburnt casings of incendiary bombs which were made of a combustible alloy, file the surface off and then pack the shavings mixed with horticultural sodium nitrate into a piece of old metal pipe. Press the contents well down and with a short spirit soaked cotton fuse set light to the whole thing, get out of the way and wait for quite a decent explosion! No one I knew personally was damaged but bad injuries were often reported. There were so many explosives and explosions occurring around the area that the odd small one was not even noticed. I was at this time a member of a local boy Scout troop and we were invited to become messengers for the local Home Guard riding around the district on our bicycles. This was quite interesting as the Littlehampton Home Guard was the nearest organisation to the Warmington-on-Sea group that one could imagine. The CO being the local accountant and very similar in looks and demeanour to Captain Mainwaring of Dad's Army fame.

Chichester was 3 miles distant from RAF Tangmere one of the most important fighter bases in the country flying Hurricanes and Spitfires during the Battle of Britain so there was much to watch. We all went to school with our gas masks in cardboard boxes for a year or so, but as the local battle faded these were no longer considered necessary.

A number of bombs fell on Littlehampton, one at the bottom of our road which killed the local church minister and his family. I remember looking out at the sky and seeing what looked like a snow storm which was caused by the church hymn books being thrown into the air by the explosion. So, the War was very prescient and possibly dangerous although as boys we found it exciting.

In 1941–1944, I slept in a so-called Morrison air raid shelter a steel table-like structure placed in our dining room. I would do my homework on the table surface and then move down below to sleep. I seldom felt frightened and despite food rationing I was never hungry but missed the odd sweets.

In 1942, the school Air Training Corps was inaugurated and as for many of us our main aim at the time was that of becoming Spitfire pilots we joined eagerly! We attended lectures and drills and an obsolete Hawker Hart biplane was placed in the main school quadrangle over which we used to crawl and sit in the cockpit to feel we were half way there. We were given an old aircraft engine on which we were instructed in basic mechanics taking it apart and reassembling it several times. On occasion, we were taken to Tangmere to see the real thing — great excitement! Marching and parades were a bore, but we were very proud to get into our uniforms.

As the war proceeded, a number of the younger Masters were called up and old and distinguished teachers were brought out of retirement. These continued to give us, in retrospect, a very good teaching experience. There was no unruly behaviour, discipline was strict and I managed to pass the necessary terminal examinations.

The main focus of the battle by 1944 had turned towards the preparations for the 'D' Day invasion. About 10 weeks before the day, our part of the coast to a depth of about 10 miles was cordoned off in an area stretching from the river Arun in the west and to the Wash in Norfolk to the east. Littlehampton was therefore included in the process and access was controlled. The surrounding streets gradually filled up with military vehicles and troops. Army lorries and tanks were being waterproofed and exhaust pipes extended to be above water level. At this time, all households were asked to billet members of the armed forces. We were asked to house the CO of the local Air–Sea Rescue base at Littlehampton located in the harbour. I was delighted by this and chatted to this man about being in the Air Training Corps. He said 'If you would like to come out on one of the Air–Sea Rescue launches, put on your uniform and it will be permitted.' Accepted like a shot!

So, on a number of occasions within a week or two before 'D' Day, I was sailing up and down the Channel seeing the preparations for Mulberry Harbour and the fleet of landing craft, etc. I was allowed to steer the boat, test fire the twin Browning machine guns and the cannon at the rear. The boats had three 500 HP engines could reach nearly 50 knots and almost outrun the German E boats. Totally exciting and much to boast about to my friends at school. My mother was not desperately keen on this idea.

The evening before 'D' Day was startling. At about 8.00 pm we heard this noise of multiple aircraft engines. We went outside and wherever one looked in the sky there was a vast Armada of Dakotas and other large aircraft towing Horsa gliders. This went on for hour after hour — a most impressive demonstration of military might. Things were actually happening at last!

Thereafter as the landings became established the focus of the war activity moved away from the south coast and the level of excitement dipped. School now began to take first place and Higher School Certificate was looming.

How all this experience contributed to my future educational prospects as a surgeon is perhaps a little dubious. Thoughts of the Spitfire pilot element quickly faded and the new school Rugby Club became our primary focus of extracurricular activity together with the usual pursuits of tennis, swimming and cycling. Female attentions had yet to divert us!

The two years in the sixth form passed quickly and I succeeded in gaining my Higher School Certificate with first MB exemption. It looked as if I was being committed to medicine and the idea of becoming a GP in a pleasant Sussex practice seemed a very reasonable life style solution. Becoming a zoologist or botanist did not appeal. I therefore applied for a place in Medical School. I was interviewed and turned down at the London Hospital and then tried at St Bartholomew's Hospital, supposedly the most difficult to get into and not being very hopeful of success. 'Barts' as it was usually referred was the oldest hospital in London founded in 1123 and possibly the most famous!

My interview was tough, one of the persons on the Committee of three was the Dean, Sir William Girling-Ball — the prototype for Sir Lancelot Spratt immortalised in the 'Dr in the House' series of books and films by Dr Richard Gordon, incidentally a Registrar at the hospital. Almost the last remark to me by Sir William Girling-Ball was 'For God's sake speak up boy I can't hear a damn word you're saying' — I've blown it!

I've had two significant premonitions in my life and I had my first as I walked out under the arch of the famous Barts Square and through the Henry VIII gate into Smithfield. Namely, I would be spending most of my life working in this place with its vast history dating back almost 850 years (see Fig. 1.2).

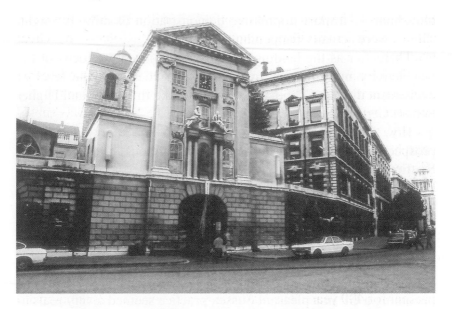

Fig. 1.2.   Henry VIII Gate, St Bartholomew's Hospital, London.

The early history of the foundation of St Bartholomew's Hospital revolves around a member of the household of King Henry I named Rahere. He was a man who appeared to have been a social climber and a wit. His name is first noted as one of the minor canons of St Paul's Cathedral in 1115. The author of this account was himself a monk and considered Rahere's life worldly and sinful. Rahere realised that he was going in the wrong direction and went on a pilgrimage to Rome to change his ways. Here, he fell ill and prayed to God to cure him and return him to London and petition the King to allow him to build a hospital for the sick poor in the City of London. He was cured, travelled back to London and had a vision of St Bartholomew that he must "build his foundation" dedicated to St Bartholomew in Smithfield, London.

Rahere duly received permission from the King and in 1123 ground at Smithfield (Softfield) was dedicated by the Bishop of London. A house was built for the accommodation of a new monastic order "The Austin Canons" and a building for the sick that The Austin Canons would administer and care for. Rahere became the first Prior of The Austin Canons and died in 1143 and his tomb can still be seen in the Priory church of St Bartholomew the Great nearby.

The hospital developed from a small hospital house and became an important shelter for the sick poor and many children in the city and became an institution of social importance. Nursing was subsequently carried out by Nuns who in due course had their own small church built, St Bartholomew's the Less, which still exists in the Hospital precinct. In 1539, The Priory was suppressed by King Henry VIII. The hospital just managed to continue but it seemed closure was inevitable. The City corporation petitioned the King to reinstate the hospital with its vital functions. In 1544, the petition was successful and the hospital was enabled to continue and a new master was installed.

From this time onward the hospital continued to develop and prosper for 400 years. The National Health Service was inaugurated in 1948 and despite later attempts to close the hospital in the 1990s it still continues as a Regional Cardiac Centre although its function as a general hospital has ceased.

Three days later I received a letter announcing I had been selected as a student at the hospital to start in September 1946. Someone was watching over me! I could not believe my luck.

I was set to go to Barts in September when I was informed that due to the large numbers of ex-service personnel being demobilised and who were being given priority access to University I would have to undertake my two-year period of National Service first. Having been in the School Air Training Corps, I was to be enlisted in the Royal Air Force.

Chapter 2

National Service in the Royal Air Force

I was enlisted as an Aircraftsman second class to be trained as a radar operator. At this time, it was not possible for National Servicemen to be trained as pilots and hold a commission in the Royal Air Force. This was because of a surplus of air crew left over from the war and still serving. My school contemporaries who had been in the Army Cadet Force were commissioned as second lieutenants, most annoying!

I started out for Padgate RAF camp in Warrington, Cheshire, in a blizzard on the 30th of January 1947. The worst winter that anyone could remember. Snow and ice lay heavily on the ground. Fuel was rationed to 5 cwt of coal or coke per month per household and my poor mother struggled to keep warm.

I had not been north of London in my life and the train journey seemed interminable and into a wilderness such as I had never experienced being the small day school pupil that I was. At Warrington station, a group of us were collected in an army lorry and taken to the camp which was a military hutted arrangement. The billets were wooden with negligible heating, bedding was two blankets, a straw filled mattress and a bolster as a pillow on an old iron bedstead. The windows were nearly all blackened out having been covered in tar on the outside as an air raid precaution. All around was much ice and thick snow.

We were due to be indoctrinated for two weeks, kitted out and then sent to so-called *square bashing* units for three months' basic training. We were still dressed in civilian clothes, mostly flannel trousers, sports coats and raincoats. There was much waiting around and we were about 30 persons to a hut. As for my colleagues I could barely comprehend what they were saying — Durham miners, Liverpool van boys, broad spoken Glaswegians, Country boys and the occasional well-dressed spiv. Quite a severe shock to the system of a Southern 'Mother's Boy'.

Between waits, we were given the task of scraping the tar off the outside of the windows with razor blades despite the fact we were still in our civvies and a blizzard was blowing. I was frozen and this was one of the lowest points in my whole life.

Over the two weeks, we were gradually fitted with battle dress, boots, great coat, etc., given medicals, inoculations and occasional lectures on what was expected of us. Food was basic and most of the time we spent speculating as to where we were going next. There appeared to be six training camps distributed around the country and I prayed to be sent to one down south which in fact happened and a number of us were packed off by train to Yatesbury a camp on the top of the Marlborough Downs near Calne in Wiltshire.

Just before leaving Padgate, an order had come round that as so many potential medical students were being called up we had to be given the opportunity to become nursing orderlies in the RAF medical service. I said 'Yes please' as I had been heading for training as a radar operator!

We arrived at Calne at night in a snow storm to find a similar hutted arrangement. Still 30 to a billet and ours run by a psychopathic corporal who eagerly joined in with the routine humiliation of the recruits a feature that seemed endemic in these institutions. The huts were less basic with clean windows and polished floors (by the recruits of course) — beds still covered with only two blankets and no sheets, but at least there were pillows.

I was selected by the corporal to be the so-called *Senior man* in the hut, probably because I could read and write and was supposed to lick my colleagues into some sort of shape — also being responsible when things went wrong. The other joy of the situation was that the bitter weather continued and there were six-foot snow drifts up against the hut walls. Obviously, square bashing was out so we had further lectures on how to take a Bren gun or rifle apart and put it together etc. Lectures on hygiene were given — appropriate because our washing facilities were a series of wash basins in a separate hut, two showers and about six toilet cubicles some without doors and above all freezing cold. Gradually, the thaw set in and we could get onto the square and were taught how to march, carry rifles, and generally behave like military automata.

Six weeks into our time, it was announced that due to the lack of heating and other amenities military camps all over the UK were being shut down and the troops were being sent on leave! A small snag — we were one of the camps that was to stay open to accommodate personnel from all the units around us which were being closed because of epidemics of either Diphtheria, Scarlet Fever or Meningitis. Patients with these illnesses were transferred to Yatesbury! Because of the risk of Meningitis, we were to keep the hut windows open, remain fully dressed, i.e., great coats, balaclavas, scarves, gloves and boots — day and night. I remember lying on my bed with snow gently blowing onto me and vainly trying to keep warm under my two blankets. We looked expectantly to the time for our first 48 hour leave pass. I went to the local phone box to inform my mother of this but was feeling a little poorly. I saw in the small mirror a completely beetroot red face. I did not care what I had but I was going to get home, so I managed to get a coach to London and then a train to Littlehampton feeling a bit more than a little groggy. I was put straight to bed, our splendid local GP was called and Scarlet Fever was diagnosed. This was quite a virulent attack and the doctor said "I would like to try a new medication on you. It's called Penicillin and has to be given by twice daily injection." This was started and was agonising. Each intramuscular injection was 10.0 mL in volume, bright yellow and was painful, so that one watched the clock dreading the next treatment. Nevertheless, it seemed to work and after five days of this medication I began to recover. Naturally, he had to inform my unit as to what was going on and did not let me return until about six weeks later. It was bliss.

Finally, I returned to Yatesbury but having now missed my particular course no one knew what to do with me 'So you are going to be a Nursing Orderly you had better go down to the hospital and find something to do.' It was wonderful as it was nearly the only warm structure in the whole camp and in an even warmer environment, I was put to running the steam sterilizers, for preparing instrumentation and dressings required in the operating theatres. After about another six weeks, I was detected and told to get myself to Marsworth, the medical and nurse training centre near Tring in Hertfordshire. No more square bashing — great!

By the time I arrived at Marsworth, the weather had improved and the six months I spent there were quite pleasant. The camp was situated on the bank of the Grand Union Canal with a nice pub adjacent. The billets were warm Nissen hut units and each accommodated about 15 persons. The bedding was civilised, the washing facilities good and the food was tolerable. The best feature was my new colleagues.

Several of them were potential medical students like myself and the remainder were very pleasant, the abrasive elements of the training camps having been sent off to more aggressive occupations (see Fig. 2.1).

Our course instructor was a likeable sergeant who took us through a complete course of nursing procedures, how to dress wounds, apply plaster of Paris, bandages, bed bathing, splinting, simple medications, invalid diets, making beds, giving an enema etc. One month we spent under canvas at a Field Hospital, lighting stoves for cooking and medicinal necessities (see Fig. 2.2). The best fatigue was to peel huge amounts of potatoes which I found restful as we could sit down and talk to one's friends as one peeled away, the sun was shining and we did not need to expend a large amount of energy.

I chummed up with another potential medical student, Tony H., who was due to go to the London Hospital as I was to Barts.

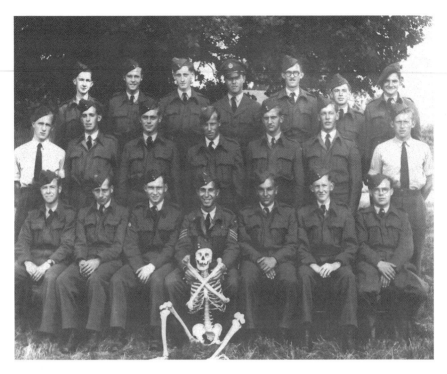

Fig. 2.1. Marsworth 1947, RAF nursing orderlies course.

He came from Woodford in Essex and had discovered a scheme whereby we could escape from the Air Force for at least some time each week. It had been decided on high that as medical students if we could do something towards our medical career, we could be given a day off for this each week. Tony had found out that we could join a suitable course in Biochemistry at the local Technical College near his home in Essex. We could have our fares and fees paid. The CO, a doctor, agreed to the plan and arranged for us to join the course. We took off early by train on a Wednesday morning to Walthamstow, attended a three-quarters of an hour lecture then an hour in the laboratory until about 12.00 pm after which we were 'FREE'. We went to Tony's house nearby, had a good lunch prepared by his mother then moved up to the West End to the cinema or a theatre. The 11.00 pm train took us

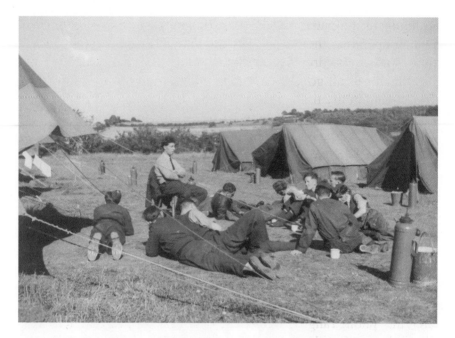

Fig. 2.2.   Marsworth 1947, mobile field hospital.

back to Marsworth — a very good day and a successful escape from the RAF for a few hours. Tony and I kept in touch for many years subsequently and qualified in our own hospitals in the same year.

It was a beautiful Summer apart from a widespread epidemic of poliomyelitis, which we luckily avoided, and the time went very pleasantly. We passed our end of course examinations and awaited our postings to active RAF units.

I was lucky and was sent to RAF Station Hospital at Uxbridge which was an old brick built facility and we lived in comfortable barrack blocks. Shortly after I arrived, the whole facility was taken over for the 1948 Olympic Games, the troops being posted out and the accommodation made available for the Games competitors, 20 or so to a barrack room. No *en suite* accommodation or individual flats as in 2012! The hospital was kept open to treat any medical emergencies.

I was allotted the job of attending to the RAF Senior ENT Surgeon, a pleasant Air Commodore. The work consisted of arranging his outpatient clinic, preparing the instruments required in a small operating theatre and assisting at any simple operations — sinus wash outs, dressing mastoidectomy wounds, cleaning ears, etc. which was all good background information for my subsequent life. I found in my time in the RAF all the medical officers, bar one who found that I was a potential medical student, went out of their way to teach me some of the basic medical processes in the areas in which I was then currently working. I had no ward work at Uxbridge and as the clinic only functioned three days a week, this was hardly arduous.

The year went on and the subject of postings came up as we were supposed to move around. Uxbridge was the Headquarters of No. 11 Group Fighter Command and I got to know some of the clerks in the posting office and I said to one person with whom I was friendly 'If you ever get a slot at Tangmere in Sussex, I would love it' being only about 10 miles from home. About two months later, the 'phone rang 'Got a post at Tangmere do you want it?' 'Yes' like a shot and at the beginning of 1948 I was posted to this very pleasant base. Incidentally, pay was increased from four shillings to five shillings a day on promotion to aircraftsman first class!

So I finished my first year of National Service despite starting with some rather uncomfortable interludes but ending up quite agreeably. I had accommodated personal relations with many different strands of society such as I had never before experienced. I had fallen in love with a charming WAAF lady of similar age but who was wholly mature beyond my years, wisely realised that I had a very long road to take before any thoughts of permanent relationships could be considered and gently led me to a sense of reality.

The Sick Quarters at Tangmere had been destroyed during the Battle of Britain bombings and was now temporarily located at what had been the medical facility for West Hampnet aerodrome — later to become the Goodwood Motor Racing Track nearby. We were about a mile from this aerodrome and 2 miles from Tangmere in a small hutted hospital complex of one large ward of ten beds and three single-bedded rooms. There was a consulting room for the MO, an office, a waiting room, a kitchen, dining room and a Nissen hut for sleeping accommodation for the other ranks. The MO lived in the Officers Mess at Tangmere and we were autonomous. The staff was the MO, flight sergeant, a corporal and six of us nursing orderlies. Quite a pleasant little team. As I could vaguely type I was put in the office to type up the medical records with very little else to do. I did, however, manage to get the whole base nearly closed down! The MO said 'We have to send a sample of the sewage plant effluent for testing to the pathology laboratory at RAF Halton. Go down to where the water flows down a stone gulley and take a Specimen.' I set off with the Unit driver to the sewage plant and collected a sample as instructed which was sent off for analysis.

Two days later there was total chaos. 'The whole station will have to be closed down immediately as there is gross infection in the all the sanitary arrangements.' I was sent for by the MO. 'Where did you collect the sample from two days ago?' I said 'As instructed where the water flows over a small gulley.' The MO said 'Come and show me!'

By now, a large penny had dropped. Had I taken the sample at the wrong place? As we approached the plant, the MO headed to the gulley. Unfortunately, this was an entirely different one at the final exit of the effluent. I acknowledged I had collected the sample as instructed but kept rather quiet as to the precise point where this had occurred. A new sample was taken and sent off for rapid analysis which proved satisfactory and the emergency abated! I did not confess there might have been some dubiety as to the point of collection of the first sample! One gulley looks much like another in a sewage plant, the detailed anatomy of which I was not familiar!

Alternate 48 hour passes each weekend and most evenings off duty enabled us to cycle down to a Chichester cinema or pub. The City of Chichester was very war weary and rationing was in full swing so food was limited and many shops were closed. The whole feeling was one of grey depression. The whole country was financially restricted. Germany was divided and France was recovering from its occupation. European travel was not possible for the majority of the British population. Nevertheless, as summer approached things seemed to cheer up as occupations such as swimming became possible. At Tangmere on one day and night a week one nursing orderly had to move to the control tower to man a small medical emergency facility and also the large Austin ambulance parked alongside in case of flying accidents. During my time, there were no major incidents that concerned me although the occasional wheels up landings occurred with two squadrons flying the new Meteor jet fighters.

The other benefit I acquired at Tangmere was that I joined and was included in the Station rugby team. This appointment involved in season a match on a weekday and one on a Saturday usually against other 11 group teams although we also competed with Army units locally or with the Royal Navy at Portsmouth. So, in season, almost two days a week were taken up for which we were allowed leave. We travelled round to other 11 group stations either by bus or flying in an old Airspeed Oxford Aircraft in which we used at other times to cadge a fun lift on short Flights one of which turned out to be more exciting than one could have wished. The first MO had been posted to RAF Wattisham in Norfolk and was being flown there in the Old Oxford. I was asked if I would like to come for the trip. It was a miserable wet day with low clouds but we got there and had a quick lunch and prepared to return. Wattisham was a grass aerodrome with no concrete runway as at Tangmere. The pilot was quite young and as we started the take off run. I looked from the co. pilots seat to see him as white as a sheet. He said "The damn thing will not take off from the muddy grass." We were heading directly towards the station buildings and at the very last moment became airborne, just avoided the building and banked sharply to miss the local church spire. We at last stabilised and flew back to Tangmere at about 2–300 ft to stay below the clouds. <u>NOT</u> a fun day out.

Most of the rugby team were pilots from No. 1 Fighter Squadron and that is as close as I ever came to flying in a Spitfire, which was packed in as a front row forward with several of the pilots and I was glad that I was not involved in any flying training!

I managed to buy an old Royal Enfield 250 cc motorcycle for £10 and petrol coupon permitted me to journey around the district when off duty and sometimes travelled home to see my mother. The second MO, also a conscript, was of a different character and finding out that I was a potential medical student let me sit in at his clinics when he taught me several practical techniques and other useful medical information. He subsequently became a Consultant Physician in Bournemouth and I met up with him at a social engagement in the 1980s and found him just as pleasant and not at all changed.

So time went on and light at the end of the tunnel in December 1948 was approaching. Then disaster again! All demobilisation was stopped because of the Berlin Crisis and the need to keep the Air Lift going. Was World War III going to start? This did not affect us directly but it meant that I had to serve for another six months and was not released until June 1949 thus losing another complete academic year. As I had already risen from AC2 to AC1 and LAC, the CO at my final interview said that if I signed on he would make me a corporal on the spot. I declined his kind offer!

In retrospect, I came to see that National Service had been a valuable experience for me.

I am sure that if I had gone straight from school to Barts I would have been very immature. My experience in the RAF[a] toughened me up considerably and having to meet, work and play often with rough and abrasive persons, certainly knocked a few of the rather delicate spots off me.

I felt in this time I had matured and could behave more like an adult and not as a school boy. I am sure it helped enormously in my medical career by enabling me to relate to and more effectively deal with the many different levels of society that I subsequently met.

---

[a] Royal Air Force Non-commissioned Ranks in 1945: Warrant Officer, Flight Sergeant, Sergeant, Corporal, Leading Aircraftsman, Aircraftsman 1st Class, Aircraftsman 2nd Class.

Chapter 3

Undergraduate Training

I had to wait until September 1949 to start at Barts Medical College, London. To give a full flavour of what it was like to be a medical student in post-war London is worth examining in detail. Each year consisted of about 60–70 students and about 50% were female. Of the men, 20% were ex-service persons who were taking the opportunity of a University placement having already achieved a sufficient educational standard. The remainder were students fresh from school as were most of the women.

It was not possible to accommodate all these persons at the College and we all had to live out and find our own accommodation. I could not afford accommodation in London and I opted to travel each day from Littlehampton by train — 90 minutes each way. There was a concessionary Fare of £16 a quarter to encourage persons to move out of London to the South Coast at this time and I managed with this arrangement for most of my undergraduate training (see later).

Having wasted three academic years, I was eager to get going and started at The Medical College on September 1st, 1949. This was sited in Charterhouse Square, London in the old Charterhouse School premises which had suffered considerable bomb damage. The subjects to be studied were Anatomy, Physiology and Biochemistry with Pharmacology.

The Anatomy Department was headed by a famous Anatomist Professor A. J. E. Cave. Our year was only the second to include female members and the Professor with a wicked sense of humour teased them considerably with remarks that by today's standards would probably get him into trouble with political or gender correctness. He lectured us about three times a week, frequently taking pinches of snuff between statements.

An introduction to the dissecting room was a jolt. We put on our first white coats and were shown into this large white tiled room the size of about two tennis courts. It smelt of formaldehyde and on display on white ceramic tables were 15–16 dead bodies supine and totally naked. Several persons had to be excused as 'feeling a little faint or slightly nauseated.' Around the corpses were senior year students working away at dissection, chatting happily. We were divided into groups of four instructed to work together and allocated to a specific body. The anatomy of the body was conveniently considered in five parts, one part for each term of our 18-month programme. These were Head and Neck, Chest, Abdomen, Arm and Leg. We started with the arm and dissected this for three sessions a week. Our four consisted of one lady and one man direct from school, one Ex-Service Pilot from the Army Flying Corp and myself fresh from The Air Force. When we were confident that we knew a specific area we sought out one of the three Demonstrators who were qualified doctors doing a period of intensive anatomical training before taking the primary Fellowship of the Royal College of Surgeons examination. These persons walked continuously around the dissecting room and when their attention had been secured we asked them to examine us on our work done on the part. They then signed a score booklet in which were inscribed marks out of ten for our effort. These events occurred five times each term. At the end of each term, all the bodies had been dissected by students at various levels of training and the remaining parts were placed in coffins and discretely taken away by undertakers for burial.

End of term assessment was by two written examinations of about two hours duration each. By the termination of the whole course, one had a very comprehensive knowledge of the whole human anatomy. A degree of knowledge that has lessened in the shorter training programmes of 60 years later.

The second major subject was Physiology, the Professor being a very distinguished scientist Professor K. J. Franklin who lectured us at least twice a week.

Practical Physiology was tame compared to Anatomy. We demonstrated the effects of nerve stimulation on recently dead frogs, blood pressure effects and drugs on anaesthetised rats etc. were tedious. We took occasional medication and recorded the effects on ourselves or partners. We did eyesight and hearing tests and tests of tactile sensation on various areas of the body and also swallowed intra-gastric tubes to gain samples of gastric contents for analysis. We demonstrated the effects of lack of oxygen on ourselves and other interesting reactions to testing the various bodily reflexes!

The Physiology Demonstrators were a different species to the Anatomists. Some were medically qualified and seemed to have given up practical medicine while others were pure physiological scientists who appeared to exist in an alternative environment. We were only examined by the end of term written examinations and not by viva interrogation unless a demonstrator casually passed by.

Next, Biochemistry — which at this time appeared a rather dry and uninteresting subject. The lectures were good but unless one was seriously interested in organic chemistry it did not appear to be particularly relevant to our ultimate goal. Little did we appreciate how critical this was to become in relation to clinical medicine in the next two decades.

My attitude to Biochemistry was a little casual during the middle two terms and my departmental examination results had been quite poor. I was suddenly jolted out of my complacency by the spectre of a likely failure in the second MB examination in the spring of 1952. I therefore settled down to read all our course text books of the time, and anything else that I could get hold of which seemed relevant. At last when the examination came, to my relief, I passed quite successfully and was runner-up for the Biochemistry medal!

Finally, the second MB arrived, some of the examinations taking place in the Apothecaries Hall in Blackfriars Lane near the hospital. Little did I imagine that 40 years later I would be in this same Hall for a rather different purpose — see later.

I managed to pass the examinations and as a result of these I was also awarded two internal Barts scholarships and was offered a place on the so-called intercalated BSc Physiology course of London University which allowed a few students to pursue a period of extended scientific study in mid-medical training. I was offered a place in the Physiology group from Barts which in fact led to one of the most valuable parts of my undergraduate training. There were three other students from Barts on this course — two men and a lady — the one I had worked with on Anatomy dissections and to whom I became very attracted!

The whole year was made up of two or three students from each of the London teaching hospitals making about 30 persons in all. The plan of the course was that we all circulated through each of the specialist departments of our various hospitals spending a week or so at each. In this way, we were taught by many of the luminaries of the time, some clinical and some purely scientific. We were taken to specialist lectures at the Royal Society of Medicine, the Royal institution, etc., and gained first-hand knowledge of the latest research going on in many areas such as the USA and South America. Especially memorable was a Professor Lorente Da No who described his method of extracting neurotransmitters from 20 barrels of ox brain. Intersynaptic transmission by substances such as acetylcholine were being studied in Cambridge. The physiology of the cerebral cortex was being worked out and the neuronal connections in the brain and peripheral nerves described. Cardiac and respiratory function was being more fully understood physiologically both from the aspects of muscular activity and neuronal control etc.

The students came to Barts to study Enzymology and it was then we began to fully understand the nature of Biochemical energy transmission and the development of the theory of the so-called *Tri Carb Cycle* of ATP, ADP and AMP, the related phosphate bonds and the breakdown of creatinine phosphate in muscular activity, etc. Most exciting and rapidly becoming relevant to clinical medicine.[a]

All this was totally stimulating and one could have spent a whole life working on just one aspect of molecular bodily functions but it was all too much detail to take in a short time as we were completing the BSc course in just eight months. I was completely diverted by the physiology of the nervous system on which I spent quite a lot of my time. We also learnt the basis of using a Scientific Library and referencing systems and were granted honorary access to the largest medical library in London at the Royal Society of Medicine where I spent a few happy hours browsing among the fascinating original volumes. We also learnt how to write and present a scientific paper with the art of referencing.

The final examination took place at the Examination Halls of the University in Kensington which were large glass roofed structures like greenhouses with no air conditioning in a very hot summer. Two other causes for perspiration apart from the examination questions! I feared the worst but was happily surprised to receive my first degree BSc in July that year 1953.

So now, back to becoming a doctor and feeling a little better educated not only in science but in life style generally. During all the degree study period, I had been commuting by train from Littlehampton, 6.15 am train up in the morning and 5.00 pm back in the evening, 90 minutes each way. Good for reading going up to London. Good for sleeping going back. Then an evening's work until midnight. It toughened one up and social life was severely limited! I could not afford to live in London but the season rail ticket costing 16 pounds a quarter made existence possible. I had ten shillings per week to buy lunch in the college dining room at ten pence per day with the occasional half pint of beer with colleagues on a Friday evening before catching the train home.

I started clinical work at Barts in September 1953 and got my first full length white coat which we wore the whole time we were

---

[a] Much practical research was being carried out at the time by Professor Lord Adrian, Professor of Neurophysiology at Cambridge who lectured us on two occasions.

students when in the hospital. These were clean and starched each week, obtained from the ward laundry cupboards and even if ignorant we looked the part and patients normally addressed one as "doctor", a big ego boost! The programme was six months surgery, six months medicine, then two years circulating through all the specialist departments.

A short description of the hospital arrangements at this time

Barts was very well organised after a major reconstruction in the 1920s and 1930s. The main hospital block consisted of a five-floor central spine with two wings on each side situated at the south side of the main square, one wing being for Medicine and one for Surgery the whole being arranged in an 'H' shaped configuration. On each wing on each floor, there were two wards of the 'Nightingale type' accommodating 30 patients, one for males and one for females. There were no cubicles or bays on the main wards which were fully open. Privacy when necessary was achieved by floor length curtains that could be pulled around individual beds. Leading off a ward entrance corridor on the right side were the sanitary facilities which were quite basic. There were three lavatory cubicles and several wash basin areas. All these arrangements were accessed by an area called 'the sluice' in which there was a large ceramic cleaning trough with hot and cold water taps above which was shelving for the storage of clean urine bottles, bed pans and washing bowls. In all, totally primitive. Next door, there was a single bath tub bathroom and a laundry cupboard.

On the other side of the entry corridor, there were two small side wards, one with one bed and one with two. Next was the ward kitchen where light dishes could be prepared for patients unable to eat the ordinary meals which came up each day in heated steel trolleys from the main kitchens in the basement.

Each whole suite was completed by an individual sitting room for each ward sister on either side of the main access corridor leading to both wards and on one side was a small lecture room to accommodate the students. Next door to this was the unit secretaries office. Quite a well thought out arrangement in the 1920s when most patients were treated in bed but quite inadequate for the requirements of post 1950s medical care when nearly all surgical patients became ambulant very rapidly.

The toilet facilities in particular were very sad, unhygienic and almost completely inadequate. Nevertheless, the patients were kept clean and immaculate by the immense efforts of the nursing staff.

On each of the surgical floors there was an independent small wing with a designated operating theatre suite.

Staffing was provided by five units so-called *firms*, five medical and five surgical each on a separate floor and distinguished by a colour. On the surgical side, these were Pink, Light Blue, Dark Blue, Yellow and Green and the medical firms had a similar but different colour code. Each Surgical firm consisted of a Senior and Junior Consultant. A Senior and a Junior Registrar and a Senior and Junior Houseman. The Nursing staff had a different hierarchy which was intimidating! Each ward was ruled by *The Sister* — who was the leader of the pack and these ranged from the younger impressively efficient and human ones to the older, fearsome and totally terrifying eminences from a different era. With the former, you could occasionally engage in an informative discussion, with the latter, one received a directive and no argument.

The Junior Nurses of varying grades were a wonderful array of attractive young ladies, so many in fact that one's eyes could not help but be distracted from the job of becoming a doctor.

All nursing staff were immaculately dressed. No evidence of a stain on white starched aprons. The blue and white striped dresses beneath the aprons were elegant as were the halo style caps — all apparently designed by Norman Hartnell the Queen's couturier. There was no make-up, no jewellery, and hair was tidy, and arranged so as not to obtrude onto the neck below the cap. Vigorously inspected on commencing duty at 8.00 am on the wards, they were expected to remain in pristine condition no matter the stress of the day. Any soiled apron was immediately replaced and hands and arms repeatedly washed. The Sisters wore long sleeved dresses with starched cuffs and a long cap known as a veil which stretched down from the head at the back to shoulder blade level. If I recall correctly each ward staff comprised the Sister in a blue dress, the deputy Sister in a pink dress, the staff nurse in a striped dress with a blue belt and silver buckle and approximately four to six nurses of lesser grades who appropriate to their year of training wore white or grey belts. All worked on a ward of 30 patients during the day time hours. The sense of discipline was very apparent.

Each day, the nurses assembled around Sister's desk near the ward entrance at 8.00 am, prayers were said, the progress of all the patients was reviewed and duties for the day allotted. The Sister then proceeded to a round of *all* the patients, talking to each and examining the temperature and treatment charts hung on the bed end to ensure all was well. In some wards, this round was accompanied by the houseman or registrar. Patients were then given breakfast mostly in bed with a few ambulant ones being served at tables set in the aisles of the ward. This was followed by bed baths for those unable to get up while the ambulant patients went out by way of the so-called sluice at the ward entrance for necessary toilet purposes. Patients were then returned to bed or to a chair by the bed and all was tidied in preparation for the Consultants round usually at 10.00 am. By this time, all appeared immaculate. Bed covers straightened, bed lockers cleaned, bed castors aligned, water glasses filled — one could go on and on with the various small tasks that were performed to keep the patients cared for and by present standards amazingly well tended.

The Consultants' rounds then took place with each patient being reviewed by the Medical, Nursing Staff and students (Fig. 3.1). This sometimes made for some very large rounds resulting in as many as twelve persons round each patient bed. An intimidating experience for the patients and making private discussions between patient and Consultant difficult. Those Consultants with insight would steer the round away from a specific bed, draw the screen curtains and engage in a personal exchange in private with the patient. All patients were visited, treatment and progress were noted and once the round had taken place, the Consultant usually withdrew with the students to the

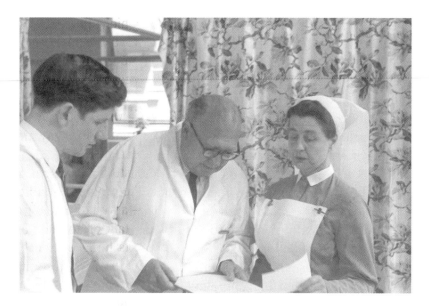

Fig 3.1. Consultant round, Mr A. W. Badenoch and Sister J. McKie.

so-called *Path room* or students lair on each floor for a short teaching session. By 12.00 midday, all medical staff and students were expelled from the ward by the Sister and lunch was served to the patients. Those too weak to help themselves were fed by the nurses. All was cleaned away by 1.00 pm and the ward closed down for rest hour. Woe betide the member of the Medical Staff who intruded during these hours except in an emergency. The fierce older Sisters were not averse to expelling distinguished Consultants who over shot their time and would pass notes to them saying Dr X please leave the ward Now!! Dr X usually departed very quickly with grovelling apologies!

By 2.00 pm, there were more Consultants or Registrars rounds in some wards. New patients were admitted and examined. Tea was served around 4.00 pm after which visitors were allowed onto the ward until 6.00 pm when they were extruded. For an hour, chaos seemed to reign as beds were totally remade and patients again tidied up as necessary. Supper was served at 7.00 pm and the ward put right by the time night staff arrived at 8.00 pm. Again, a discussion followed around Sister's desk to appraise the night staff of events and necessary treatments. The ward gradually quietened and lights went out at 10.00 pm after an evening drink. No television of course. Wireless earphones were allowed for some.

The night shift of usually a staff nurse and two to three junior nurses then took over and supervised late drinks and settled all down. The night Sister who was responsible for a number of wards usually made her first round between 10.00 pm and midnight and checked for any problems, all was hopefully tranquil. Her second round was usually at about 5.00 am to 6.00 am but she could of course be called at any time of emergency. The night Sisters were usually older, very experienced and always managed to control minor problems. With obviously difficult situations, she would call the Houseman. If called by night Sister it was as well to get to the ward at once because this was usually a serious problem especially if Sister had presented her compliments to Dr X and 'would he attend the ward at once!' There were no pagers or telephones and the message was brought to the Houseman's bedroom by one of the outpatient porters with a Sister's note pinned to the patient's note chart and treatment board.

This brief resume may, I hope, give some impression of nursing and ward life as I remember it as a Medical Student in the 1950s which I trust is not too distorted.

The young nurses were of course an enormous distraction for the testosterone loaded young student gentlemen of the time. There were many sly glances, winks and smiles exchanged and romances blossomed. It was an extremely difficult task to arrange an assignation with a young nurse in training. At work from 8.00 am to 8.00 pm with may be a rest from 2.00 pm to 4.00 pm in the afternoon in the nurses home. This establishment was strictly supervised by the Home Sisters and effectively limited any hanky-panky. No male person was allowed in the nurses home! Occasionally, in this building which was known as 'The Virgins Retreat,' dances took place under the eagle eyes of the Senior nursing staff. Off duty amounted to one day per week when the nurse was allowed to emerge from this quite severe regime and unless journeying home or on holiday had to be back at the nurses home by 10.00 pm. The number of strategies developed to work around these restrictions is another story! Fortunately, I was somewhat protected from these hazards by my attachment to my medical student colleague already mentioned above!

The Firms were conveniently arranged so that each had its own "duty day" on the same day each week and every fifth weekend when emergency patients were dealt with either in Casualty or on the wards where a few beds were kept vacant for unexpected admissions.

When I returned to the hospital, I was directed to join the Light Blue Surgical Firm. The Consultant's name was displayed above each bed and the patient knew exactly who was responsible for his or her case. The Chief of this Firm was Mr J. P. Hosford, tall, always elegantly attired with neatly brushed hair, moustached, with a spotted bow tie and a dark suit was then regarded as technically one of the best surgeons in London. Mr Edward Tuckwell, the Junior Consultant, a very kind and friendly man, always smiling and dressed in a more tweedy country style, was also the Dean of the Medical College and well-known for his speed of operating. 'He's come back before he's been' was applied to him and as I frequently heard him referred to.

There were eight of us on the Firm with about 50% being female students. From each of the Surgeons we were given a ward round a week, plus other sessions with the two Registrars. We were allotted about four patients in each ward to whom we had to introduce ourselves and after asking permission we took a history and examined them under the eagle eye of the Ward Sister and other Nursing staff. We then wrote up our notes and findings on the treatment board hung at the foot of each bed which accompanied the houseman's own notes and the drug chart and temperature chart. Each patient had a small wooden locker by the bed for personal effects and privacy when required was obtained by the eight foot curtains which could be pulled round the bed. These were always drawn when we examined the patients.

On the Consultants ward and teaching round, we had to read out our notes to the assembled company and which were then taken apart, congratulated or criticised as appropriate. Some Consultants taught by gentle humiliation others by gentle encouragement i.e., remarks on the students notes such as 'a pedantic old man of 42 years' raised a few laughs from the Consultant. Another old gentleman who also caused amusement all round and who had a rather red nose and scarlet complexion who had vouched to his embarrassed student that he 'hadn't touched a drop for 30 years.' All carefully recorded by the student who had then described him somewhat inaccurately as teetotal! Some patients who were obviously seriously unwell were not taught upon.

On the surgical firm, we attended the operating sessions of the Consultants and Registrars when our designated patients were undergoing a procedure. We were also allowed to scrub up and hold retractors and other instruments.

First time in theatre was intimidating, our dressing and scrubbing procedures were strictly controlled by the Theatre Sister or Theatre Superintendent, the latter being a fearsome lady with much experience of dealing with awkward students. We did not change completely but wore our ordinary clothes covered by a sterile gown coupled with hat, mask, rubber gloves, white clogs or rubber boots. We found standing for an hour or so at the operating table was onerous and occasionally resulted in someone passing out. This was quite an obvious sequence before the event the sufferer first turning pale, then green and then hitting the floor. Total collapse was normally short circuited by the theatre technician being called by Sister to help Mr So and So to sit down and have some water. The grim message was 'do not under any circumstances fall into the wound!'. We were usually taught at the operating table and just watching the proceedings was interesting and only occasionally boring. At this stage, I was perhaps beginning to feel a slight attraction to surgery as a future occupation!

We attended three of the six months in the related outpatient clinics both pre- and postoperative. On the Firms duty day which occurred on the same specified day each week we attended Casualty and saw patients needing admission to our related wards. Life was quite packed and there was much text book reading to catch up with in the evenings. I still commuted to Littlehampton! As we were closely involved with the firm, the Consultants got to know us as individuals and I was amazed that even as a student in subsequent years one would occasionally be greeted in a hospital corridor and addressed by name.

For the next six months, we were directed to the Medical wards of the hospital in the George V block. I was attached to the Medical Firm of Dr Spence a small avuncular, gregarious gentleman who practised in the whole spectrum of General Medicine while Dr Oswald, the Junior Consultant was tall, elegant, and also the principal Chest Physician of the hospital.

Ward rounds occurred as in surgery with two consultant rounds each week from Dr Spence who taught us the intricacy of cardiac medicine and how to auscultate the heart. We developed a "journey-man's facility" in Cardiology and learnt why the stethoscope was called the "guessing tubes".

There were a number of rounds on patients with various hormonal disorders, a speciality of Dr Spence with thyroid deficiency such as myxoedema or thyrotoxicosis with excess thyroid hormone. Cushing's disease was noted together with other problems with over or under active adrenal glands. Pituitary disorders such as acromegaly were also demonstrated. Diagnosis and the control of diabetes featured prominently as various new preparations of insulin were just being introduced. The problem of gastro-intestinal ulceration was common at this time. There were usually one or two patients in the wards being treated by a purely milk diet administered by an indwelling nasogastric drip. Gastric haemorrhages were quite frequent and occasionally required surgical control by operation. To witness a patient having a severe gastric vomit of perhaps a pint of blood or more spread over the bedclothes and floor was quite alarming and induced a feeling of helplessness in the observer, especially as some bleeds were lethal. Another welcome to the actual practice of medicine.

Patients in severe cardiac failure were nursed in chair beds so that their legs were dependant and often grossly swollen. To relieve this accumulation of fluid small stab incisions were made all down the legs to allow this excess fluid to drain into rubber sheets and be caught in large galvanised baths. All this is now controlled by medication. In other words, we were given an excellent grounding in the major medical conditions we might come across in general practice.

Dr Oswald of course dealt in detail with various respiratory conditions. At that time, the classic London "Pea Soup" fogs occurred regularly. I clearly remember in 1954 the literally "Green Fogs" which completely shut down the City of London. They were so severe that I recall standing at the ward door, totally unable to see more than half way down the ward — the further patients disappearing from sight into the green/grey distance. The conductors on buses had to walk in front of the vehicle and guide the driver with a torch and I remember getting completely disorientated on my short walk from Blackfriars tube station to the hospital and having to feel my way along the front of buildings which I normally passed each day. These fogs of course brought in with them bouts of bronchopneumonia and patients frequently died in the wards of respiratory failure.

Pulmonary TB was also quite common as the anti-tuberculous medications such as PAS and Streptomycin had only just arrived. All these conditions produced asthmatic or respiratory symptoms which Dr Oswald specialised in treating. Patients were kept on oxygen masks or in oxygen tents as ventilators were not in common use at this time.

We also attended the relevant outpatient clinics and the X-ray department to learn how to interpret simple chest and abdominal X-rays. The art of angiography or the demonstration of the patients vasculature had not been developed at this time and it was impossible to demonstrate if blockages had occurred in the coronary pulmonary or carotid arteries. The Physicians were entirely different in their demeanour in contrast to their Surgical colleagues. I began to feel Medicine was not quite my scene but supposed this was all part of the medical process one had to absorb. There seemed little we could do of a 'hands on' nature and I guess I was slightly bored. The days of active interventional medicine had not arrived and it seemed all one could do for patients was to diagnose and prescribe medication then wait often for very prolonged periods to witness any therapeutic effect. The months passed slowly and I was anxious to move on to the specialist departments where we were not attached to specific Firms. Outpatient clinics were also attended. There were firm parties at the end of each six-month period before we moved on. This medical firm was well recognised for its hospitality and Dr Spence's parties were not to be missed especially as he was known to enjoy a fair consumption of the refreshments. The parties were held in various areas of the hospital and it was the duty of the students to make sure that any medical staff who succumbed, would be suitably returned home by transport and delivered to their front door!

So all in all a very pleasant six months during which I was certainly taught many useful features of the general medical scene which I found invaluable in later practice when some odd unrelated conditions presented themselves!

The Specialist Departments then Started

Ophthalmology

Firstly, a short period in the ophthalmology department was stimulating because the surgeon in charge was Mr Hyla Stallard who had been a Gold Medallist runner in the 1924 Olympic Games. Mr Stallard was tall and lanky and never appeared to stand still. When we had to follow him around the hospital, he used to semi-run. The main difficulty was stairs. He appeared to ascend these by taking the steps about three or four at a time followed by an exhausted team of students.

His primary interest in the eye was intra-ocular tumours and he used a method of treating them by radiation, placing a radioactive plaque on the back of the eyeball, a treatment that is still occasionally used today. We were of course taught the normal testing of vision with letter charts, looked for colour blindness astigmatism, detection of squints, retinal diseases and the prescription of spectacles. We also learnt to examine the eye with an ophthalmoscope, etc. We did see some action in the eye theatre, but nothing at first hand — a pleasant and restful period!

Dentistry

The Dental Department in the outpatient clinic was interesting because of its interventional aspect. In other words, we were trained to extract teeth. Here, we attended a lunch time clinic where patients scheduled for extraction were lined up. usually about six persons. The patient was placed in the dental chair and an anaesthetic mask producing a nitrous oxide/oxygen mixture was applied. When the patient was suitably unconscious, we were allowed to approach with the dental forceps and hopefully arrive at the affected tooth. A good grip was obtained and with a comprehensive twisting, yanking manoeuvre which if successful allowed extraction. Various events followed if this was not achieved. If the patient was still asleep, the dentist moved in and the tooth came out. Sometimes, a student was allowed to have a second go. If the patient came round and the student was still using the forceps a struggle would occasionally follow with the patient being heaved out of the chair on the end of the forceps and attempting to fight off the operator. On rare occasions, all contestants were known to finish up on the floor with the anaesthetist trying to gain control of the situation and all frequently getting covered in blood. As students we thoroughly enjoyed being involved. What the patients thought and experienced is better not recorded. Conservative dentistry seemed a long way off and we were not allowed to attempt tooth filling!

Anaesthetics

Anaesthetics was another interventional subject in which we were allowed to carry out procedures at first hand. We attended various operative procedures in different theatres in the main hospital block. Anaesthesia was going through a period of rapid development. Intravenous administration of Pentothal, a barbiturate for primary induction had recently been introduced, which allowed a more pleasant and calming way for the patient to be rendered unconscious. Once asleep, the normal respiratory anaesthetic was administered by way of a nitrous oxide, oxygen mixture. Ether was added as necessary and was still widely used especially to obtain good muscular relaxation for various surgical procedures. This, however, took a long period to clear from the body postoperatively and gave rise to most of the unpleasant well-known effects of nausea and vomiting. Other gases were being trialled such as Halothane which cleared from the body very quickly with less unpleasant symptoms. Chloroform was rarely used because of its cardiac-toxicity. Short acting barbiturates and curare type relaxants were being talked about, but little used at this time. These of course finally changed the whole field of anaesthetic medication. Endotracheal intubation had not been commonly adopted and a simple mouth airway and mask was normally used and held in place by the anaesthetist.

We injected Pentothal, applied the masks and waited for the patients to sleep and then under the eye of the anaesthetist we sat with the patient throughout the operation usually holding the mask on and watching and adjusting the gas supply as necessary, but now sitting down and seeing more varied surgery than had been viewed when on the surgical firm.

Anaesthetists were of differing temperaments from the 'jolly good fun old boy' to the depressives who spoke little and never smiled, especially one who existed with the appellation of "Gloomy" known throughout the hospital. A recorded minority were 'sniffers', i.e., those who derived satisfaction from the intermittent inhalation of their own "gas" mixtures from the masks. These were usually taken care of by the theatre technicians who gently reapplied the mask to the patient having removed it from the anaesthetist and no one seemed any the wiser (see later). So much for health and safety!

Psychiatry

So to Psychiatry. These lectures were some of the most stimulating of my undergraduate training. The head of the department was a very distinguished clinician Dr E. B. Strauss who was author of several books on the subject. His description of the various disorders was graphic, almost theatrical and made the subject come alive and to make some sense. He was always immaculately dressed with a bow tie and accoutrements. The most fascinating eccentricity was his hairstyle. His hair was somewhat sparse but he had trained a few stray strands and wound them around the back of his cranium and somehow secured them horizontally in an attempt to give some ground coverage but with a rather unconvincing result. This feature riveted the eye of the beholder when he turned to face the blackboard followed by a very piercing look on facing the front again for anyone who had produced a snigger. We had two trips to mental hospitals in the periphery to see the various conditions at first hand. A number of my contemporaries were so stimulated at that time they considered the possibility of a career in this speciality which did not particularly appeal to me as a way of life.

Neurology

The Department of Neurology was headed by Dr J. W. Aldren-Turner, a most gentle and polite physician, who taught us the basis of neuropathology and its various manifestations. Having had my neurological interest aroused during my period in neurophysiology for BSc, I was eager to learn how this knowledge could be referred to the clinical situation. Unfortunately, the answer appeared to be very little at this time apart from its anatomical element as an aid to diagnosis.

Most clinical neurology appeared to be dedicated to the amelioration of the after effects of intracerebral vascular accidents of various types. If the patient survived a stroke, the treatment seemed to be related more to physiotherapy or re-education than helpful medication. Another area of activity was multiple sclerosis and its derivative effects. There seemed little of therapeutic assistance that was available and that could be effective. Epilepsy was another subject area treated by variation in medications — some effective, some of little help similarly Parkinsonism. It was at this stage I became disenchanted with the thought of a career in pure neurology which offered an interesting diagnostic and intellectual exercise but little of practical utility to the patient. Much more was to follow later!

Dermatology

On we went to Dermatology with Dr McKenna, a very pleasant and friendly clinician. The wonderful array of rashes and itches affecting the population seemed endless. Obviously, a Contact Dermatitis could be improved by avoidance of the primary irritant which seemed logical. Psoriasis seemed common and responded very slowly to treatment. A number of dermatological manifestations of general medical conditions were enlightening and worth remembering in later years of medical practice. A vast menu of medications were available for treatment ranging from lotions through creams and ointments to ultraviolet irradiation. If one does not work, try another! I left impressed by the old adage on the dermatological process 'Dermatological patients never get better, but they never die.' Perhaps, a little unfair but not far from the reality.

Orthopaedics

Orthopaedics was an interesting speciality. The acute admissions came by way of Casualty and comprised dislocations and fractures. We were instructed in the necessary clinical examination and X-ray assessments of patients. In orthopaedic outpatients, we learnt how to reduce dislocations of the limbs and the re-alignment of fractures and plaster of Paris splinting which always for no apparent reason involved a period of frivolity. Why this should be I cannot in retrospect conceive. Major trauma such as fracture of hips, fractures or dislocation of the vertebrae were of course major events at which we could only gather round as observers. Osteomyelitis was quite common and treatment with the new wonder antibiotics was just commencing. Failure to respond often resulted in amputation.

Arthritic joints were treated in various ways. Some were excised and the bones re-aligned. Some were arthrodesed (stuck together). There were also occasional amputations. Replacement of arthritic hip joints with artificial prostheses was just beginning to be experimentally investigated and I do not remember any such operations being performed at this time. One could always tell in which theatre "orthopods" were performing by the noise of whirring electric drills hammering and peals of laughter.

Many of the dislocations and fractures were sports related injuries and the male orthopaedic wards seemed populated by otherwise active young men who were full of life and testosterone much to the embarrassment and enjoyment of the junior nursing staff but a cause for anxiety for the ward sisters who seemed to spend an amount of their time installing some sense of discipline into a rather rowdy party atmosphere.

We attended a few orthopaedic lists but took no part in actual procedures. I was left with the final impression that the subject was a rather rollicking specialty led by a team of merry extroverts! Manipulation of patients limbs and spine was a revelation. Patients would be put in apparently judo-like holds when the various portions of their troubled anatomy were seized and stretched and pulled into amazing configurations. The operation notes would record such words of wisdom as 'two good cracks obtained' or similar!

Paediatrics

Next on the list was paediatrics, taught by an important and knighted paediatrician — Sir Charles Harris. His teaching at the bedside in the children's wards was crisp and didactic. Patients' relatives were plainly informed of their child's illnesses and what was to be the plan of treatment if any. Being a specialist unit in the treatment of childhood leukaemia, the prognosis in many cases was bleak with numerous early deaths. The children amazed me, for even when seriously ill they remained alert and active until shortly before death. The Ward Sisters really were angelic both with the care of the children and the management of the relatives which obviously took up much time. They never appeared rushed or impatient and I admired them tremendously. We did little practical work in the unit and could only get a brief history of the child's condition usually from the parents if present and examination was only carried out when indicated on a teaching round. The children did not appreciate the attention of another apparent doctor and were frightened that this meant more painful blood tests or other discomforts so we stood well back and observed. I remember thinking that paediatrics was definitely not for me.

Ear Nose and Throat Surgery

Ear, nose and throat (ENT) patients were quite interesting. We were allowed to look down throats, ears and nasal cavities with an interesting number of instruments — some of endoscopic design. We tested hearing with tuning forks etc. but did no practical therapy and purely attended lectures and the theatre sessions where I can remember what seemed a sanguineous progression of bleeding and screaming children who had undergone tonsillectomy quite often six or seven in a row!

Social Medicine

To be given a background of social medicine, we were taken in small groups by district nurses to visit the various housing facilities around the Hackney and Islington areas. We visited private dwellings and were always well received by the residents who seemed very willing to show us around. We saw how babies and children were cared for and the way in which the households were managed by housewives who seemed to me as a young medical student prematurely aged. The uniform seemed to be a wrap round floral apron and a headscarf. We saw small businesses being run from ground floor workshops mostly concerned with furniture making and repair. These were currently under pressure from larger multiple firms which were now taking over this activity. The families lived above often in obvious conditions of near poverty and where there was evidence of the terminal effects of the recent bombing raids of the 1940s. I was consistently struck by the cheerful friendliness with which we were received, especially when we were introduced as young doctors from Barts!

Another memorable visitation was to the newly established St Joseph's Hospice in Hackney developed by Dr Cicely Saunders who over the next many years went on to become the most important initiator of this type of facility all over Britain.

I was amazed by the care and obvious contentment of the patients mostly suffering from terminal conditions such as cancer or cardiac failure. Dr Saunders and her team of devoted nurses and carers were doing a truly marvellous and necessary job but received little government funding at this time and relied almost entirely on voluntary local support and the occasional legacy to survive.

Gynaecology

Our near final session was devoted to Gynaecology and Obstetrics. Gynaecology was taught by three different surgeons. The most senior was an older and very distinguished man, Mr John Beatie, who spoke softly and treated the lady patients with great politeness and gentleness and was obviously much appreciated. Ward rounds and outpatient clinics were conducted in a narrative manner with little in the way of hands on examination for obvious reasons of decorum. Pictorial representation of the female anatomy was by photographic slide display.

The second gynaecologist was a little more racy in his attitude. He addressed all his students as 'My darlings' and patients were treated similarly. His raciness extended to his personal dress which tended towards the 'bookmaker' mode with check suits with flower buttonholes and yellow waistcoats. To top it off, he drove a red drop head E. Type Jaguar (just out) which was reputed to have been described by his Senior as 'that motorised pessary'! His outpatient sessions and ward rounds were conducted with a degree of hilarity which eased tensions all round and were much appreciated by the students if not always by the patients.

The third surgeon fell between these quite different attitudes and was pleasant, informative and taught well. Quite a spectrum to choose from, but we were certainly 'well educated' by the time we had finished in this part of the hospital practice.

Obstetrics

Then came Obstetrics where we probably became more directly involved in the medical process than in any other part of our training.

Obstetrics as a student

In obstetrics, we were instructed in the delivery of babies which we performed if the birth was not too complicated. Two months were allotted to this, one on "the District" at Barts in which we 'lived in' ready to be called for home deliveries and one Resident at Rochford Hospital Southend with in hospital deliveries. The aim was to achieve a total of 30 deliveries.

The district was the most exciting and occasionally a complete eye opener. A delivery in a Peabody apartment in the East End of London was more than socially instructive. If memory serves right, each was a single room about 20 ft long and 8 ft wide. The entry door lead onto a communal balcony walk way. On the right side of the door was an old stone sink with a cold water tap. On the left side was a simple table with two chairs.

Towards the back of the room, on one side was an iron range with a smouldering fire, a blackened kettle on top and a cupboard and at other side a bunk type bed and chest of drawers. The flooring was linoleum or tiled. The toilet facilities were communal and at the end of the outside open walkway.

We always met with the local midwife at the time of the delivery. She would instruct and take over if necessary and take care of the baby. Frequently, there was a grandma, husband or even other children around at the time of the event which was usually over very quickly and the baby placed in one of the drawers of the chest. A cup of tea was our usual reward.

On another occasion, I was called to a woman in labour in a flat in Hoxton. This was on the upper floor of an old Victorian terraced house. I arrived by bicycle at about 3.00 pm. The labouring mother was lying in an ancient iron bedstead with very scanty bed clothes. The floor of the room had once been covered in linoleum which was now blackened and wrinkled. I was welcomed by Grandma 'Good afternoon doctor this won't take long, it's number 6!' She drew up a chair close to the mother and said "Sit there dear you will get a good view" then proffered a brown paper bag and said 'would you fancy a whelk?' I politely turned this down and the bag was then offered to the labouring mother who said 'no thanks I don't feel quite like whelks just at the moment.' A small child of about six years old then arrived 'Ere' said the mother feeling under her pillow for her purse 'Ere's two bob, go and see your bruvver — he's in the Fever Hospital.' The two bob was pocketed and he disappeared. No sign yet of the midwife and apprehension set in. I was chatting quietly with Grandma when there was a sudden commotion in the bed — a few grunts, a swishing noise and a baby's cry. We rapidly peeled back the bed clothes to reveal a healthy number six. I was just getting myself together again when the midwife arrived and took over! 'Thank you doctor' says Grandma 'that was easy wasn't it?' Shortly after the small boy arrives back chewing. 'You ain't been to see your bruvver? You've spent that two bob on sweets — push off.' We then all had a 'nice cup of tea' and I had somehow clocked up another delivery! Just like 'Call The Midwife.'

We then went to Rochford Hospital near Southend for one month. At Rochford Hospital, deliveries were "in house" and we also attended the outpatient clinics which were interesting for the number of unexpected and illegitimate pregnancies that seemed to roll in. Apparently, the Southend district held the National record for this type of activity. The patient usually greeted the news with a little dismay when the diagnosis was confirmed. The lady consultant dealt with this by a slap on the stomach and by saying 'Don't worry dear go off and get married and we'll tell your Mum it was a bit premature!' The other excitement was the extroverted Obstetric Registrar who drove a Sunbeam Alpine sports car between the two hospitals Rochford and Southend and gave one a lift saying 'I never drop below 40 mph including roundabouts it is such a bore.' I survived and finally achieved my 30 deliveries total.

Another little annoyance is worth recording. At Rochford Hospital, the call system consisted of 2 ft strips of illuminated coloured lights on the wall in each part of the accommodation. Everyone was given a code and if one was required this appropriate colour code flashed up on the lights. Viz. my own code was red flashing, blue static and yellow flashing. If this code showed you rushed to the nearest telephone to see where you were required. The drawback was that you had at all times to watch the lights to see if it was your code being presented. You could never sit quietly having a meal, writing at a desk, or watching television as you constantly had to look at the lights to see if it was your code. This resulted in a sort of 'light twitch' and indigestion. I have never encountered this system at any other hospital.

Forensic Medicine

We were now coming towards the end of our general training. The cherry on the cake was Forensic Medicine! In this, our instructors were two of the most famous Home Office Forensic Pathologists of the time. Professor Keith Simpson and Professor Francis Camp who had been concerned with some of the most notorious cases of criminal activity of the 1940s and 1950s and whose names and photos appeared regularly in the daily press.

The forensic lectures were the most well attended of the whole medical course as the lecturers presented graphic details of poisoning, battery, rape and murder and the manner in which forensic methods had brought a large number of very nasty persons to justice and even death by hanging still existent at that time. The two men were again in entire contrast. Dr Simpson was tall, urbane, good looking and always elegantly dressed in a dark suit. He spoke quietly and succinctly and seemed to treat the whole gory business quite factually and non-chalantly. Dr Camp on the other hand was in strict contrast. He was short and stout and addicted to flowered waistcoats with a gold watch chain across them and a buttonhole in his black jacket. His descriptions of the various cases were vivid and dramatic with students on the edge of their seats awaiting the next ghastly detail of some foul crime but all told with a dash of humour. Greatly appreciated by the audience. We were fortunately not taken to the crime scenes!

Pathology

Apart from all the details of purely clinical activities described above we also attended lectures and demonstrations in clinical bio-chemistry, macroscopic and microscopic tissue pathology and bac-teriology usually in the afternoons.

Biochemistry

The biochemistry course was related to tests of normal levels of blood constituents such as the electrolytes, sodium, potassium, chloride, etc. Organic constituents such as albumen, globulin, urea, creatinine and tests related to the normal function of the liver, kid-neys and endocrine glands were also studied.

Haematology

A second section was devoted to haematology and the varying lev-els of the different blood cell constituents, the red cells, white cells, platelets, protein levels, etc. both in the normal condition and dis-ease demonstrating abnormalities of cellular production and the cellular response to infections other pathogens and cancers.

Histology and Postmortems

Whole organ and microscopic pathology entailed trips to the museum to examine preserved specimens of various diseased organs in glass jars. The museum contained one of the best displays of pathological bits and pieces of abdominal human tissues in London (Fig. 3.2).

There were examples of the largest and the smallest everything on record. From the largest bladder stone or liver tumour or the longest tapeworm discovered in the bowel or the smallest skeleton, etc. One of the most studied sections was that of foreign objects recovered from various organs, such as a cannon shell of 2.0 inches in diameter removed from a patient's rectum or the ball point pen removed as well as an open safety pin from a urinary bladder and the rather large stopper from a thermos flask removed from a patient's vagina, used as a contraceptive. All these articles having been reportedly introduced accidentally caused enormous if not lethal trouble and were usually related to some deviant sexual practice, the cannon shell being described by the patient as the instrument that he frequently used to reduce his prolapsed piles. The glass tumbler open end downwards introduced into the rectum proved quite a problem but was solved by eventually filling the glass with a plaster of Paris bandage which was allowed to set solidly and the whole then removed by a good firm yank on a tail of the bandage left outside.

It was a pleasant environment to while away a happy hour and frequently very illuminating. Incidentally, a small room off the museum was designated The Sherlock Holmes Room, reputedly where Dr Watson and the Great Detective had their first meeting.

This was coupled with regular attendances, usually daily at lunch time, to the postmortem room when newly deceased persons were examined and the pathology of their demise scrutinised and discussed in detail, occasionally in enough detail to spoil one's appetite for a good midday meal.

Microscopic sessions were regularly held to observe the effect of various pathologies at cellular level such as the nature and natural history of the differing types of cancerous growth and other evidence of distorted cellular mechanisms. Occasionally, some abnormal piece of tissue or insect might be introduced to a fellow student if known to be of a squeamish nature, delivery being either on the hand or by way of a shirt collar.

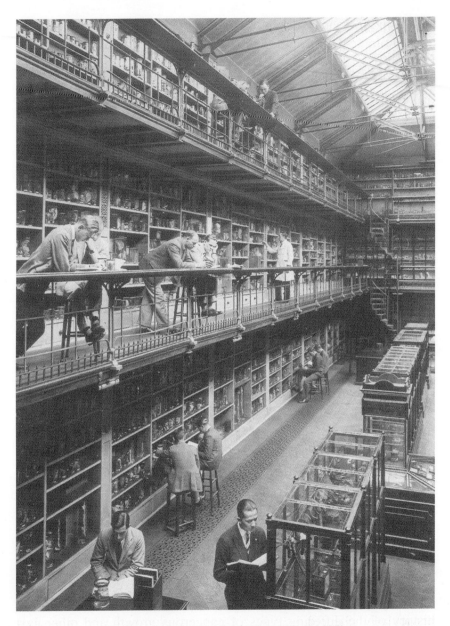

Fig. 3.2.   Pathology museum, Barts Hospital 1950.

Bacteriology

Bacteriology was an entirely separate subject and encompassed the growth and incidence of the many pathological bacteria surrounding us coupled with the resultant disease pathology that they produced. The various species of bacteria were identified microscopically, cultures were grown on agar plates and the activity of antibiotic agents and their effect upon the different organisms studied and correlated with the clinical syndromes which they produced. Other pathogenic organisms, etc. were discussed such as tics, scabies, bedbugs, etc. The immunology of cellular defence mechanisms was studied such as vaccination and the administration of vaccines against small-pox and other virus infections. We stood well back from some of these potential pathogens and the importance of hygienic handwashing was engrained. No one developed a transmitted disease that I was aware of.

These lectures were conducted by the very distinguished bacteriologist Professor L. P. Garrod, one of the pioneers in the study of antibiotics. All these ancillary studies took place alongside our clinical commitments and entailed endless note taking and textbook reading so there was little time for social activities especially as I was still making the long train journey each day. My friendship with my co-female medical student was thus rather strained and meeting up was especially difficult but of necessity our relationship cooled somewhat.

The Beginning of the End

In the autumn of 1954, the day of reckoning arrived with the advent of the final Pathology Examinations. These appeared to be quite reasonable and I was happy to get a satisfactory pass mark.

Revision lectures and ward rounds now took place. I was not particularly cheered by one Consultant Surgeon who remarked 'I don't know why you are bothering to take this examination Wickham. It is so obvious you know little surgery.' Such remarks stimulated one to get out the textbook for the third time of reading.

As the spring of 1955 arrived, examinations in the major subjects of medicine, surgery, gynaecology and obstetrics came upon me. Each exam comprised two 3-hour written papers, a practical exam and a viva. These latter two events took place at other London teaching hospitals so there was no chance of getting away with a friendly chat with persons one knew and the written papers were all marked by external examiners. The whole arrangement was spread over four to six weeks during which one's adrenaline level was exploding through the top of the head! The London University degree Bachelor of Medicine and Bachelor of Surgery were regarded as the toughest. One could try for the Conjoint Diploma of the Royal College of Physicians and the Royal College of Surgeons which was recognised as being somewhat easier. If you were really stuck you could go for the Licentiate of the Society of Apothecaries which also granted a licence to practice medicine.

My recollection of these few weeks is sketchy. I only clearly remember my practical Medical Examination at University College Hospital when I was examined by one of the most famous Cardiologists of the time. I was asked to examine a patient with a heart condition and fumbling with my brand new stethoscope I listened exhaustively to the patient's heart and to my horror could hear nothing abnormal. The examiner arrived and said 'Well what did you hear?' I owned up that I could detect no abnormality 'Neither can we' he said and I nearly fainted. Next patient please.

The great day came when the results of the examination were published as a list on the metal gates of London University at Senate House in Bloomsbury. With leaden heart and ulcer pain, one stepped up at 5.00 pm to the list surrounded by crowds of students from all the London teaching hospitals.

At last, I found my name on the list. I had passed. I was a doctor. I don't think I have ever had such a surge of relief in my whole life. I phoned my mother from a call box and said "This is Dr Wickham speaking" and she burst into tears.

So ended six years of rather concentrated sweat, anxiety and cerebral exhaustion. Incidentally, my girlfriend passed as well and we celebrated over a cup of coffee in a local café.

If I had known what was to follow I would have looked for that GP practice in Sussex straight away!

Time Does Not Stand Still!

Having qualified the next vital step was to obtain a house appointment. One had to serve in one of these appointments for a full year to obtain full registration to practice with the General Medical Council. The most sought after jobs were at Barts and about a half of each qualifying year were successful. I applied but did not get a one year general appointment but had put my name forward for six months neurological surgery to continue my interest in neurology. I was successful and was appointed to the neuro-surgical house job at Barts temporarily located at Hill End Mental Hospital near St Albans to where 200 Barts beds had been evacuated during the war and were awaiting repatriation to London in new accommodation. My new chief was Mr John O'Connell. A solemn man in his demeanour. He was known subversibly as laughing John O'Connell.

Chapter 4

House Appointment at Hill End Hospital, St Albans Herts

I arrived there at the beginning of July 1955 having been picked up by my new chief Mr O'Connell in Finchley Road early one morning. He, living in London and driving to St Albans every day, kindly offered me a lift. It was intimidating having a close discussion with my first chief at 7.30 am for three quarters of an hour! On arrival at the hospital he deposited me at the hospital residence. I was shown to a large very pleasant and comfortable room on the first floor of this old Victorian building. The room overlooked the front lawn which was partially laid out as a tennis court. There was a wash basin in the room and a communal bathroom along the corridor. I changed and put on a clean long white coat, grabbed my stethoscope, pen and notebook and tried to look like a doctor. I descended to the ground floor and was directed to the Neurosurgical Unit in Ward FC which was a considerable distance from the residency along several of the long bare corridors found in the old type of mental hospital. A number of mental patients were drifting along the corridors in various stages of dress and weirdness. Some smiled, some glared and one tried to grab my stethoscope from my pocket — rather different behaviour than that in the corridors at Barts! But something one rapidly became used to.

I arrived at the Unit office and introduced myself to the secretary and the then Senior Registrar Tony Andrew. The Unit consisted of Mr O'Connell as Consultant, Tony as Senior Registrar and myself as Houseman with a total of about 25 beds. Twenty beds were in a male ward and five were in a separate female ward plus two side rooms which were clearly padded cells, originally for the incarceration of disturbed mental patients.

There was a small ward office where I was introduced to a young Barts sister, Audrey Lester and her deputy. The ward appeared very busy and Tony suggested we should make the early morning round. I was delighted to see all the nursing staff wore Barts uniforms.

The patients were a mixture of postoperative and recent admissions, many who had or were going to have cerebral surgery. Some postoperative patients looked well but others were barely conscious. Tony examined them all carefully and gave instructions about treatment to Sister or the appropriate nurses. It seemed that postoperative patients who had had cerebral surgery needed and had to be checked daily to make sure that their postoperative cerebrospinal fluid had not reached serious levels of excess pressure by palpation of their craniotomy incisions. If swelling was detected then the patient was scheduled for lumbar puncture drainage. Usual checks on BP, blood pressure, etc. were made and noted. The nurses reported on general responses such as ability to eat and mobilise or not and so on. Tony said to me "you will be in charge of the lumbar puncture procedures — have you done one?" Done one! I had never even seen one or been taught one. "Okay" he said "I will show you how to do it." I was petrified. The instrumentation was brought by a nurse. The curtains were pulled round the patient's bed and he was moved onto his side with his legs drawn up to his chest. His lower back was cleansed and Tony put on a pair of sterile surgical gloves, palpated the patients lumbar spine, carefully counted the spinous process of his lumbar vertebrae 'make the puncture between L3 and L4.' He picked up a small needle and syringe filled with local anaesthetic and injected about 5.0 mL into the indicated area. Waited a few moments and then picked up a 6-inch fine needle and gently pressed it into the indicated area, advanced the needle until he felt a little resistance 'the ligament over the vertebra' and then with a final quick thrust pushed the needle into the spinal canal. At once, clear cerebrospinal fluid gushed out and was caught in a kidney dish held by the assisting nurse. After about 30–40 mL was drained, the needle was withdrawn and a temporary swab and dressings were placed on the puncture and the patient was laid flat again. The craniotomy was checked for pressure and all being well we moved on. Tony said 'By tomorrow you can do some!' I nearly fainted on the spot!

Now we moved onto the new admissions. Tony studied the outpatient documents and X-rays and said 'we will now do a full neurological examination.' I had superficially read about this in my text books but was amazed by the extent and the rapidity with which the whole procedure was carried out. Full examination of the cranial nerves, sense of smell, visual acuity, visual fields, eye movements ophthalmic examination of the retina, sensation of face and head to touch and pin prick. Examination of ears, hearing tested with a tuning fork for sound, sense. Muscular movements of face, tongue and throat. Then onto the body, chest, abdomen — arm and leg reflexes, abdomen, sensation all over the body and limbs. Standing if possible, gait on walking — it seemed endless. Tony said 'every patient gets this on admission — your job and of course regularly postoperatively as necessary. All must be written up.' I was reeling. 'Also, don't forget to talk to and explain everything to all the new patients and assess their general fitness for surgery, prescribe medications pre- and postoperative. Do ask me if you need advice!! The nursing staff will be very helpful.' Each examination took at least 10 minutes and had to be recorded in detail later. Similar examinations were carried out on postoperative patients if necessary to assess function and progress.

At last, after an intensive hour and a half, we paused for a quick cup of coffee with Sister in her office and it was then time for Mr O'Connell's round — again, he greeted each patient and there was a meticulous review of all postop patients — questions were asked and answered both ways. J. O'C, as he was called by all except to his face, was formal and reassuring and would re-examine a patient if necessary.

Finally, it was time to discuss the new patients and examine them again. J. O'C carried out his own neurological examination discussing his findings with Tony, occasionally asking me a question which I answered with some trepidation. We at last finished at about 12.00 pm. J. O'C took off and Tony said 'time for lunch.' Sister said 'Would you please write up the pre-meds and check the consent forms.' I did this at a gallop and finally got to the dining room at about 12.30 pm.

Lunch in the residency was promptly at 12.30 pm. Much to my astonishment all the Consultants, Registrars and housemen ate together. I was suddenly thrust into very close contact with several of my previous teachers from my general training who had always appeared superior, remote and from a different planet. It was totally unnerving to find myself sitting next to a Consultant Cardiac Surgeon and being asked to pass the salt or asked where do you come from? etc. 1.45 pm came and it was off to the operating theatre.

The operating theatres at this hospital were three in a line converted from old store rooms. These were neuro, thoracic and orthopaedic units, some with communicating doors between them. Theatre no. 1 was neurosurgery. We all changed into theatre kit. The patient who was due for a craniotomy for a cerebral tumour was anaesthetised and placed in a low sitting position on the operating table. The anaesthetist was entirely calm and the theatre sister was a very pretty girl! J. O'C after at least 10 minutes' washing and scrubbing of hands and arms proceeded to clean the patient's scalp with multiple washings of an antiseptic solution. Tony and I already gloved and gowned now stepped in to apply the surgical drapes and J. O'C returned fully gowned. The operation began and continued in complete silence. A scalp flap on the shaven head having been previously marked out was incised. Bleeding controlled and on being raised the flap was wrapped in moist swabs and laid back like opening a coffee jug lid. Points were marked on the cranial bone and then a hand held brace and bit was used to drill out four large half inch holes in the bone around the line of incision. The bone chips were preserved. The underlying dura was carefully separated from the bone by a flat spatula-like instrument then a wire Gigli saw was passed between one hole to another and the bone sawn through. This was repeated at each site and the bone fragment finally freed, raised and removed. The dura was then incised along the incision line and placed back against the skin flap in a moist swab. The brain was now exposed. J. O'C identified the tumour area and very gently excised it with diathermy as completely as possible with careful retraction by Tony and removed it. All oozing vessels were diathermised until the area was completely dry. The dura was then closed and the bone returned and wired in place with the bone chips placed in each hole. The wound was closed with small drains. It is easy to describe but the whole procedure took about three to four hours during which I stood patiently, occasionally being allowed to pass an instrument and keeping out of the way of J. O'C and Tony. This sort of procedure was carried out each time a head was opened either for a tumour or a bleeding aneurysm. Physically tiring as we all stood, but totally absorbing!

John O'Connell operated in complete silence and was seldom perturbed. Next door was the orthopaedic theatre where as usual there was raucous laughter, banging, drilling, sawing, etc. emerging much to his annoyance, otherwise all was silence. One day during an operation a junior nurse pushing a trolley into theatre lost her balance, shot forward and crashed into the operating trolley scattering all the instruments. The noise and disruption was unbelievable and we waited for the explosion with bated breath. J. O'C at the table looked round and made his remark of the morning 'Don't make a habit of it nurse' and carried on operating. The current operation finished, J. O'C departed and Tony and I dressed the wound and the patient left the theatre.

Tea and sandwiches were in the rest room and at last I was able to speak and ventured to address the rather attractive theatre sister who likewise had hardly uttered a word during the whole procedure. Life returned somewhat to normality. I said 'do these procedures always take place in silence?' 'Yes John O'Connell likes it that way.

We all know how he operates and don't need to communicate verbally. Okay when you know what to do but a bit difficult for the new boy! That's why John O'Connell *hates* the new houseman that he gets every six months. You know you are okay if he speaks to you after a month otherwise further silence means disapproval.' Great!

No more sitting around — back to normal. Meet ward sister to hear any news and then do another round to check up on everybody usually to about 7 pm. Examine new admissions, prescribe medications — a quick dinner then back to the ward to write up operation notes and new admission notes. Leave ward about 9.30–10.00 pm to the common room, get introduced to ones contemporaries, swap some experiences — have a cup of tea, coffee, chocolate. Final trip to ward about 11.00 pm then bed. Phew! With luck, no calls until morning. At 2.00 am, called to the ward to a very sick and terminally ill man aged in his 40s. Screens around the man who is groaning and crying out on seeing me 'Dr, you can't let me die, I'm too young to die, I have a wife and young children.' Other patients sitting up awake to see how the new boy would manage the night. No idea what to do. Young new night sister, her first time on night duty in tears at the bottom of the bed. All I can do is hold his hand and wipe his forehead. He finally relapses and dies about 3.00 am. Both the night sister and I age very rapidly and I felt that I at least was now becoming a proper doctor and not just a smart theoretical student. If this day represents medicine then I doubt that I can cope with it! Back to bed and restless till about 7.00 am when it all starts over again.

And so the six months at Hill End continued with the same format. The other major drama in theatre during these six months was the day of the ants. Hill End at that time was unusually hot. That summer was particularly so and this heat engendered a plague of Pharoh's ants — small red insects. They got into everything — clothes, beds, food, all over the hospital.

We were getting to the end of an operation and as usual John O'Connell asked for the insufflator to spray the wound with fine antibiotic powder. He aimed the spray, squeezed the trigger and outshot the powder accompanied by about six or seven live ants who scrambled all over the opened brain. These were quickly grabbed with forceps and removed and the whole area thoroughly cleaned. Tony and I were consumed with smothered laughter. John O'Connell was livid. We made feeble remarks such as 'do you think we need more drains than usual to let out any strays sir?' 'What if they get on the cranial nerves?' The patient may suffer from flashing lights and ringing bells etc. John O'Connell was not amused. P.S. The patient did well.

As a second job, I had the task of looking after six eye patients flat on their backs for days or weeks with retinal detachments. They frequently needed catheterisation because they couldn't pass urine. A tedious nuisance but new technique learnt and it was nice to chat to these patients who were not seriously ill but rather incommoded by their retinal problems.

On Christmas Day, the turkey lunch had just been served when a patient went into respiratory obstruction. The curtains pulled and an endo-tracheal tube was inserted by way of the nose. The patient takes a big breath and completely inhales the tube into the trachea. Quick thinking suggested a tracheostomy. In approximately the correct place, I made an incision, opened the trachea and recovered the tube before the Christmas pudding was being served. Another technique is learnt! And rather proud of myself for the quick recovery of the tube. A Christmas Ward Entertainment was expected of the House Staff and we tried to oblige. Somehow, I was induced to perform a Cossack Russian Dance dressed in suitable attire and white operating theatre boots. This was to the sound of a gramophone recording of a rather vigorous Russian Dance . This was reasonably well received but resulted in total exhaustion and enormous haemorrhagic bruising to both my legs from feet to thighs which took several weeks to reabsorb! I needed the exercise!

During the six months, there were endlessly long operations for the approach to the brainstem for excision of tumours on the acoustic nerve taking sometimes six to seven hours! The patience exhibited by the whole team was exceptional from the anaesthetists and all the nursing staff. This was surely the way that surgery should be conducted — a feeling which never left me even after nearly 40 years in action.

Unfortunately, patients frequently died; this was a high risk activity — about ten during my term of office. John O'Connell was very put down when he found me in the office signing death certificates and cremation forms first thing in the morning.

During my incumbency, I became slick at intravenous intubations and lumbar punctures. I became used to patient management and I hope developed a professional behaviour. During this time, I got very chummy with the pretty Theatre Sister, an affair which lasted a few months then fizzled out due to distance and intensity of work in subsequent appointments. One can only cope with one source of excitement at a time.

I had very little time off being the solo Houseman in the unit and on one occasion I did not leave the hospital for three weeks. One Saturday, I needed to go to St Albans for a few bits, like toothpaste. It was quiet on the ward and I persuaded one of my colleagues, the thoracic Surgical Houseman to hold the fort for two hours. Got back 'All quiet?' 'Was called to your ward as one of your patients had gone unconscious. Had a look but as most of your patients were unconscious I did not worry.' Shot to the ward like a scalded cat to do a quick lumbar puncture! Two weekends off in the six months I was able to nip home. Tony as cover.

We were served tea and sandwiches on the lawn on sunny Sunday afternoons and managed to fit in a quick game of tennis with other Housemen and nurses. Felt like living in a play by Noel Coward!

Other memories of this time come back. Sister on the Orthopaedic ward an imperious lady and Doyenne of Barts Sisters called Aggie and who weighed in at about 16 stone. I had to go to the ward for something one lunch time. Aggie descended on me like a meteorite and in a very loud voice echoing around the ward 'Mr Wickham *Leave my House Immediately, It's Lunch Time!*' I left with tail between my legs, and with patients and nurses sniggering.

The Sister on the Thoracic ward was the complete opposite. She was small and gentle and carried tablets of Morphia or Pethedine loose in her apron pockets and walking round the wards passed these out to patients like sweeties. 'Here you are dear, this will cheer you up a bit.'

Tony Andrew the Senior Registrar had managed to purchase a smart sports car a Triumph TR2 of which he was very keen to show off. This was a two seater with a parcel shelf behind. One evening after Dinner, Tony announced I am going to the cinema in London anyone like to come? Three persons including myself said yes and after arranging suitable cover squeezed into this small car. We shot off to the Odeon Leicester Square and arrived in 35 minutes (the traffic was a little less congested in those days) saw the film, visited a pub on the return journey and were back at the Hospital by 11 pm. The ride was somewhat invigorating! So life was not all dull at Hill End.

My colleagues were a great bunch. We covered for each other if possible but the nature of the specialities precluded much direct involvement in the various techniques required. If kept up late at night we used to finish off with a game of poker or canasta. I was very sorry to say goodbye to them all at the end of six months.

In summary, this period was a very rapid and intense human and surgical baptism. It was hard, enjoyable but rewarding work, often very tiring. I performed little practical surgery and I had never used a scalpel except for the tracheostomy but I learnt a number of very useful small techniques.

Most importantly, I think that at last I was glad that I became a doctor because I like patients. The work went on but at last I could behave more like a doctor with hands on responsibility for patients well-being and not just as an observer in the wards. In practical surgery, I had little direct experience but observed plenty and saw how meticulous procedures should be performed. I began to get a feel that I liked the idea of the direct action in surgery — long, long way to go before I could personally partake in such activities.

Clinical integrity I learnt abundantly from John O'Connell. Neither before nor since have I seen a doctor who took such scrupulous care of his patients as exhibited by his tireless attention to them in ward and in theatre. J. O'C was a bachelor at that time and it was said that he had no time to fit in a marriage — immediately after retirement, he married a Barts Sister and lived happily in Hampshire fishing on the River Itchen. He taught me clinical integrity in spades a bit of which I hope I picked up and which often guided me over the succeeding 40 years.

The Second House Appointment

Having applied for a major year house appointment at Baits without much hope, I was astonished and overjoyed to be offered the post of House Physician to Sir Ronald Bodley Scott then (currently) Physician to Her Majesty the Queen. Now I would really learn some medicine as distinct from surgery although part of this appointment was an obligatory three months as House Surgeon to our opposing Surgical Firm — Mr R. Corbett and Mr A. W. Badenoch. I have already indicated how the physical arrangement of the main hospital blended nicely with the so-called 'Firm' system both in surgery and in medicine [Fig. 4.1].

In surgery, I was firstly to join the Green Firm of Mr Corbett and Mr A. W. Badenoch for three months' surgery to be followed by my

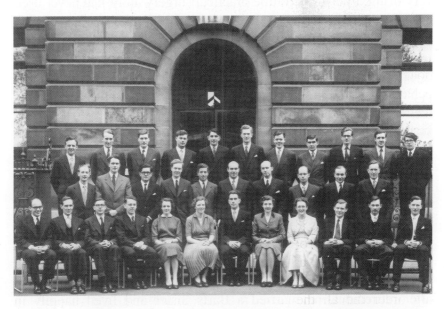

Fig. 4.1. House surgeons and physicians, St Barts, 1956.

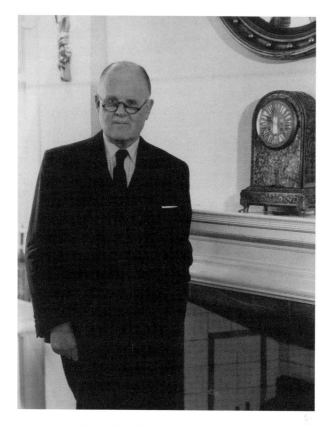

Fig. 4.2.   Sir Ronald Bodley-Scott.

nine-month appointment in medicine with Sir Ronald Bodley-Scott [Fig. 4.2].

So to three months' more surgery

The team that I was allotted to was headed by Mr Rupert Corbett, a very distinguished older surgeon about to retire [Fig. 4.3]. The Junior Consultant was Mr Alec Badenoch practising exclusively in Urology. The Senior House Surgeon and I at the bottom of the pecking order did all the usual tasks, examining all the patients on admission, doing ward treatments as necessary. I was principally

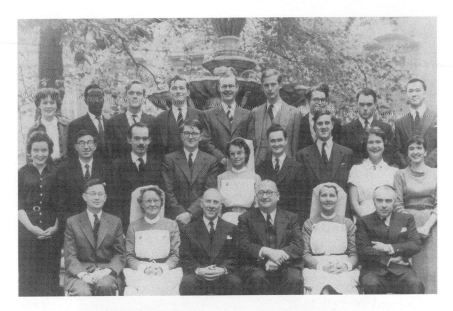

Fig. 4.3.   Green surgical firm, Mr R. Corbett, 1957.

working for Mr Badenoch and I arrived back at the hospital to start work on a Sunday afternoon in January 1956 to be greeted at the ward by a very small but fierce Sister. Mr Badenoch's main list was on Monday each week and my first question to Sister was 'What does Mr Badenoch like for his patients preoperatively.' Answer 'You're the doctor you should know.' Good start, but gradually settled down with the preop patients.

Mr Badenoch was a stout and very amiable physician who always conversed most pleasantly and never talked down to his junior staff and never directly admonished mistakes. He just exuded a slight aura of displeasure when events were not to his liking. As was usual at Barts, he was always totally polite and understanding with his patients all of which tended to rub off on his assistants.

Monday morning started with the Senior Registrar round 8.30 am–9.00 am. Mr Badenoch's teaching round at 11.00 am. Lunch, if lucky at 12.30 pm. Theatre at 1.00 pm until 5.00 pm. Now I was really able to plunge in and assist at a large number of operations with the Junior Registrar as first assistant. When Mr Badenoch had finished, the registrar and I would carry on with small operations, hernias, varicose veins, etc. until 6.00 pm–6.30 pm.

On other operation days if I had time I worked in theatre with Mr Corbett who was also the complete gentleman to patients and staff. We first met on a Tuesday morning. He welcomed me to the firm and then said 'I am due to retire very shortly. In the three months that you are here I will try to teach you all the surgery I know.' He was as good as his word. He said 'come to my list tomorrow.' I arrived and he said 'Ah, good first case is an inguinal hernia. I have just got to make a phone call — you start off.' Now for the very first time I was to wield a scalpel but I soon realised to my horror that my practical surgical expertise was nil! Where to make the incision, how long, what do you do when you have to cut through the skin? Nerves shattered but soothed by the kind anaesthetist and the delightful Sister. The anaesthetist said 'You make the incision about 1inch above the inguinal ligament about 2–3 inches long.' The Sister then passed me a scalpel and I made a feeble scratch on the skin. No evidence of an incision. 'You must press harder' Second go — not very successful. 'Much harder' I finally produced an incision. 'Now what?' Sister: 'Here you need a self-retaining retractor' and stop the bleeding. From the anaesthetist 'Now look for the hernia sac and mobilise it, open it, reduce the bowel and close it an so on.' The operation proceeded at a snail pace — where was Mr Corbett?

Finally, under dual remote control, the operation was nearly completed and Mr Corbett arrived just as I was putting in the skin stitches. So began my distinguished surgical career. The patient survived.

Over the next three months, Mr Corbett patiently took me through a number of procedures. Appendicectomy, removal of gall bladder, hernias, varicose veins, partial cystectomy etc. With Mr Badenoch, I was instructed in simple examinations such as cystoscopy and assisted at prostatectomy and the occasional renal stone operation.

Being the Junior House Surgeon, one faced two personal problems: The first being the fact that the post had no residential accommodation facility. Obviously, I could not go back to commuting to Sussex.

This difficulty was faced by all Junior Housemen at the time. We all therefore had to more or less 'live off the land' we could sleep in on our Firms duty day. We were off duty on alternate weekends when I could get home for two nights. On duty weekends, we had accommodation for the three nights required. We therefore had a number of nights when we had to scrounge accommodation. The Senior Housemen all had a room in the residents quarters so if one snooped around one could often borrow the room of one of these chaps (all men!) for the nights when they were on holiday or off duty a sort of hot bedding! Usually, this worked well but on occasions one was stuck. You then had to appeal to friends who had flats or rooms nearby and who would let one sleep on their settee etc. In general, this worked reasonably well and one was not actually on the street. Eating was also a problem but if one was friendly with the night staff nurse on one's ward you could usually scrounge a poached egg or something similar in the ward kitchen. One had of course to dodge the Night Sister!

I would perhaps mention that our salary at that point was £375 per annum now the equivalent of about £6700 per year. If we moaned about this to our chiefs the usual reply was that it was 'an honour to hold a house job at Barts and that payment for this privilege had only begun with the start of the NHS in 1948.' It was also interesting to note that until 1948 the Consultants were not paid and performed their duties as a charity and made their living in private practice. The better you were at this the better your recompense which was a splendid incentive to work hard. A factor which in the course of time has escaped the attention of some of the present fully employed and paid staff and may perhaps explain some of the attitudes of doctors who now fail to fulfil their professional obligations, for their recompense arrives whether or not they exert themselves — see the daily press!

The second problem of being the Junior House Surgeon was on the Firm's duty day and duty weekend when one was deployed for the whole of the time on duty in the Casualty Department. It now seems unbelievable that at this time during the day there were only four doctors on duty in the whole of Casualty. Also, only two Junior doctors were on night duty when the Casualty registrars went off at 5.00 pm until 9.00 am the following morning. It was not uncommon for the Junior Houseman on our Firm on duty day which was Friday to come on at 9.00 am on Friday morning and be on call night and day until 9.00 am the following Saturday morning. On our duty weekend, one could be responsible in Casualty from 9.00 am on Friday until 9.00 am Monday, both day and night. So much for the working time directive! This was medicine and what was expected of one as a doctor.

The surgical Casualty room or 'box' as it was called consisted of a room about 20 × 40 ft in area, three slots where patients on stretchers could be accommodated behind curtain screens on one side while around the other walls there was a line of about 20 chairs for ambulant patients. There were two of these boxes, one male, one female joined by a narrow corridor on one side of which was a wooden platform also screened by a curtain where patients brought in dead could be accommodated until the undertakers or pathologists arrived to collect them. To move from male to female box one had to squeeze past this slight hazard. Not always occupied, of course. As the sole Houseman, one had to cope with this mass of people sometimes of up to about 30 patients at a time if we were very busy. One had to rush from one to another examining fractures, lacerations, boils, children who had swallowed coins or pushed peanuts into their noses or ears, foreign bodies in eyes, etc. Abdominal pains were put in storage behind the screens until able to be moved to the wards! The chaos was occasionally unbelievable.

One had to perform a sort of triage. Fractures to X-ray then to the fracture clinic to be plastered if possible. Lacerations to the minor operating theatre. Two or three patients were stock piled until one could suture them. Boils were lanced here as well. Children were taken to the children's ward for treatment. Women in labour were smartly packed off to the Obstetric Department. Porters and the nursing staff were superb. All were directed by a short rather plump Senior Casualty Sister. This lady appeared somewhat menacing and directed everything like a military campaign. She had a heart of pure 18 carat and had really seen it all for many years and had an answer to any problem. Kind to the patients, tough to the staff who always sought and got her help. She really held the ship together.

If one became overwhelmed one could in day time call for help from the Casualty Registrar if available. At night, one appealed over the phone to the Firm's Senior Houseman to come and give a hand if not engaged in theatre. It was often quite difficult to get any sleep, but the porters were very good and stock piled the patients if not urgent to allow one to rest or sleep for two hours at a stretch, one slept fully dressed. Being next to the General Post Office, one of the irritations was the odd postman who would drop in at 3.00 am for a check up on his backache which he had had for four years!

We were not particularly troubled by drunks as the city closed down at night time. If we had any difficulty with such patients a quick call to Snow Hill Police Station just around the corner usually resulted in the rapid appearance of two 6-ft plus city policemen who would whisk the patient away 'Been troubling you Doc? Come along Sonny!'

One of the most impressed and sustained memories I have of this time is the performance of the Salvation Army. When one was faced at 2.00 am with a homeless patient who had little wrong with him or her apart from their vagrancy and did not require hospital admission, we were stuck. One could not just push the patient onto the street. I was told by one of the porters 'just ring up The Sally Ann and explain' I did this on a number of occasions and within 30 minutes or so one or two totally sympathetic persons would arrive and take complete care of the person saying 'We can fix you up with a bed and some food, come along.' It was this sympathetic understanding of a total social outcast that I saw at first hand and what these good people did and forever after it was the one charity that I wholeheartedly support and still do. They never failed to respond while the primitive Social Services of the time frequently promised to ring back but never did.

I really felt that I was becoming able to cope with a number of problems simultaneously and competently in a situation that no amount of theoretical knowledge could equip one for. We had little previous instruction and were dropped into the deep end. No bad thing as this vastly improved one's competence and we were doing a job that mattered at last. Again, it was very 'hands on' and one became quite adept at suturing and the appliance of plaster of Paris splints. But as far as development of practical surgical ability was concerned, there was little chance.

The following three months as a Casualty House Physician helped stoke my enthusiasm for a surgical career. Acute medical emergencies were usually admitted to the ward as soon as possible but one was occasionally allowed to perform an electrocardiogram, almost a novelty at this time and prescribe a limited number of medications, no CPR or defibrillators! Acute asthma attacks or severe epileptic fits were very worrying to manage and often required that the Firm registrar on duty be called to help out. Luckily, no deaths occurred on my patch but were occasionally a near thing.

To return to my inpatient activities with Mr Badenoch. On a normal Monday list, I witnessed my first nephrolithotomy (kidney stone removal). Having seen John O'Connell at work when the spilling of 2–3 mL of blood was almost a disaster, the contrast between this and a conventional nephrolithotomy was amazing.

Mr Badenoch commenced by making an eight-inch incision in the patient's loin. Blood spurted around and the bleeding skin and muscular vessels were secured with artery forceps and ligated. The kidney was eventually exposed and mobilised from its fatty bed. The main renal feeding artery and vein were dissected and the first assistant was then asked to compress them between thumb and fingers to arrest the circulation. A scalpel was then taken to the back of the kidney, a long incision made and the whole organ was laid open completely as for grilling. The stones were rapidly picked out of the drainage system and then large 'through and through' sutures were passed through the meat of the kidney so as to bring the two halves of the kidney back together again like closing a book and ultimately looked similar to the tied up weekend rolled sirloin. Compression on the vessels was released, the circulation restored with the average loss of about 200–300 mL of blood which oozed from the large incision in the kidney which was then sucked out and mopped up with swabs. When bleeding had ceased apart from a small ooze from the incision in the kidney, it was replaced in its bed and the wound closed in layers with two very adequate drains which continued to ooze for some time. The whole procedure was over in about 35–40 minutes. Blood was replaced by intravenous drip and the patient returned to the ward.

I was absolutely astounded. Moreover, 2–3 units of blood lost plus a large incision purely to remove a few small pieces of calcified material from an internal organ. It was the gross contrast between what I had seen in Neurosurgery and this major operative spectacle alerted me to the fact that surely there must be a more delicate way of achieving the aim of what was the conventional mode of treatment at this time. At that moment, I first felt an inkling that there was possibly room for surgical improvement in this situation but there was obviously a very long furrow to plough before I could have a go at something myself! At the end of my three months, I had learnt much and had actually got my hands albeit somewhat tremulously on the practical feel of the surgical process.

I now moved to my nine months' stint in General Medicine. This was obviously way off the surgical track and one had to assimilate an extremely different take on the clinical process. The most notable change was the length of exposure to each facet of ill health. In surgery, the clinical process is generally quick and episodic. The patient has a finite condition which in most cases is amenable to a one-event therapeutic situation. There is removal of a lump, unobstructing a blockage or stemming a haemorrhage which can be conveniently and usually dealt with in a short time period, the patient moved on and all being well is not seen again. In medicine as I mentioned above, many conditions were long in development and required a complex and prolonged detailed diagnostic process. Further was the fact that in the end treatment, usually by medication, was often slow and by oral means which achieved very long drawn out results for both for patient and doctor. Each situation might be gradually resolved but it revealed to me the rock bottom of the medical versus the surgical diagnostic and therapeutic process. The mind-set required to be a successful physician was entirely different. In both situations, it was vitally important to develop a sympathetic relationship with an ill patient. Whether you were treated by the pill or the knife, the doctor was the person in whom you placed your trust.

In medicine, I learnt by inference rather than by direct instruction from my mentor Sir Ronald Bodley-Scott. 'Always listen to the patient. Engage with them and do not brush off their queries. Reply in a polite and sympathetic manner and try to explain a situation and how it is to be managed.' I had even in my short experience seen a number of occasions when pomposity and failure to treat a patient as a sensible sensitive human being was to say the least hugely regrettable. It was by imitation inculcated into us that you were to be the helpful friend of the patient and not some bullying technocrat. A lesson that appears to have been sadly omitted in many of the botched clinical episodes reported daily in the press.

Sir Ronald was at this time the Physician to Her Majesty the Queen. He was an imposing presence dressed in a black jacket and pinstriped trousers, white shirt and discreet tie. He had a gentle pleasant voice. He was modestly overweight and progressed slowly around the wards always giving adequate time to the patients history and problems. He would assess, examine a patient and then move on round the ward. A few moments later, he would suddenly pronounce on the patient he had seen about 20 minutes ago and pronounce the diagnosis and treatment. This was obviously due to a quiet and probably complex thought process going on but rather disconcerting to the Houseman or Registrar in attendance. In time one became used to this progression.

So the nine months passed rapidly and busily. Monday to Friday up at 7.00 am, on the ward at 8.00 am, registrar rounds. Consultant teaching rounds at 11.00 am, case conferences, then writing up the patients notes and requests for investigations took one frequently until midnight. Social activity contrary to that portrayed on television was almost non-existent! Current programmes record a fantasy life with ridiculous medical situations, nurses decorated like models apparently concerned more with their social life and sex rather than their patients. I have never before or since been so tired in all my life as I was at the end of my house appointments.

At the end of this 18-month period, I began at last to be able to differentiate between the trivial and the significant, and gain some sense of proportion in the clinical process. One commenced the house appointments with a head full of textbook minutiae and rare diagnostic possibilities which although recorded were very seldom encountered — common things are common! 'Furtwangler's syndrome' may be, noted in a textbook and be on the internet list of diagnostic possibilities but will rarely be met with in practice. May be, one case in 30 years while you will have met and treated 150 or more cases of bronchopneumonia or gastric ulcer.

This ability to recognise the 'frequently met with condition' from the rarity gradually emerges by experience on the ground and explains why a purely computer presentation is so frequently misinterpreted by the beginner or the lay person. Dr Google has a long way to go to catch up with the 'time-served' medical experience!

I felt that I had finally achieved a reasonably solid base of clinical practice but with a long way to go yet before being fully competent in many areas! The call of surgery gradually became stronger for as well as its intellectual content the pace of its practical manual activity was calling me.

Sir Ronald appeared to approve of me after a while and could not have been more kind. For example, he always did a Saturday morning ward round and one day at the end of this said to me 'What are you doing for lunch Wickham?' 'I shall eat in residents quarters as usual, Sir.' 'Perhaps you would care to lunch with me at the L'Etoile in Charlotte Street?' A quick arrangement for a colleague to cover for me and I was whisked off with Sir Ronald in his Bentley. I was somewhat overawed by the initial conversation but was soon made very much at ease. This situation occurred on a subsequent occasion and at another time I was invited to dinner at his house in Harley Street for an excellent meal with his family. I always felt I did not quite achieve the same standard of social commitment with my own Housemen. At the end of my appointment, he gave me an excellent reference ending that his only regret was that 'I was abandoning a career in medicine for one in surgery.'

So to seeking another appointment was now financially essential as I was supporting my mother in our rented accommodation in Littlehampton and once household expenses had been dealt with there was very little equity available. My other grandfather, my mother's father, was very supportive at this stage.

Socially, time as a Houseman was very restricted. My medical student to whom I was attached was appointed to house jobs in other more distant hospitals and was equally busy and we slowly drifted apart. She ultimately became a Consultant Gynaecologist and we inevitably moved in other directions.

Chapter 5

The Anatomy Demonstrator

It was now time to move on if I was to seriously consider a career in surgery.

The first step entailed gaining the Fellowship of the Royal College of Surgeons. This was a two-stage procedure, firstly requiring one to achieve the so-called *Primary Examination* principally in Anatomy plus a little Physiology and Pathology. The best way to achieve this was to obtain a post as an Anatomy Demonstrator in a University Department of Anatomy. This already existed at Barts in the Anatomy Department at Charterhouse Square which I had already experienced as an undergraduate.

A job was advertised, I applied and by some miracle I was appointed and moved to the Anatomy Department on January 1st, 1957 with no break in my employment. Little did I realise at this stage the enormous significance of selecting surgery for the rest of my professional life!

When I started in the Anatomy Department, Professor Cave told me that the appointment was for two years 'The first year you are useless. The second year you might be of some slight assistance.' The job was Heaven after the house appointments! Start at 10.00 am, finish at 5.00 pm with an hour for lunch, extensive holiday breaks and a five day week! And at double the salary! I now reverted to daily commuting from Sussex as I could still not afford separate

London accommodation. The compensation was that I had three hours a day on the train for reading my anatomical texts.

The job entailed patrolling the anatomy dissecting room for periods of an hour or so at a time when one was supposed to answer questions asked by the students, help them with their dissections and examine their comprehension of their work to make sure they knew what they were supposed to have learnt from the process. This was all very well in theory, but the practicality was nerve racking. Firstly because one had forgotten the anatomy that one had learnt five years previously, secondly because the senior students probably knew more than you did and thirdly because the standard of knowledge you were supposed to exhibit to the students was initially on the zero side of negative.

One soon learnt to rise to the challenge with a few 'gamesman' like well chosen phrases "well of course each muscle/nerve, blood vessel, etc. can be very variable, keep on looking and I will return later if you are still confused." A quick nip to the demonstrators room and a frantic thumb through Gray's Anatomy enabled one to swan back to the dissecting room after a few minutes and blind the students with your new found knowledge. As time went on, one got quite good at the job, but the Professor would occasionally drop by and tease you with a tricky question. Between whiles, we three demonstrators were supposed to carry out our own dissections in the demonstrators room on specimens required for the anatomical museum next door. The whole atmosphere became quite relaxed but the doom summons to the Professor's room came at 5 minutes to five most evenings. His secretary would pop her head round the door to our room 'The Professor asks if you would care to join him for a cup of tea.' To turn the invitation down was obviously not politic and one knew an hour or even more would be occupied but not lost for the Professor always carried on a monologue of interesting anatomical tit bits and anecdotes of past colleagues and their doings. He was also the world authority on the comparative anatomy of the White Rhino and his rooms were littered with bits of Rhino in jars or on the bench raw. The Professor was also good for slightly risqué anecdotes which he would tell with his loyal, long suffering and elderly lady secretary sitting in the corner typing away and totally non-reacting to some of his more outrageous statements! Finally, we would be released.

It is now almost unthinkable but the Departmental winter dress code was overcoat, Bowler hat and rolled umbrella. We all looked like guardsmen in Civvies. The Bowler hat was a pain and got in the way of everything but was relinquished in the summer!

The appointment being for two years at double the salary of the House Jobs enabled my mother and I to look around the Littlehampton area for a new house as the rented one in which we lived was required by the owner. We found a new development in Rustington, Sussex, about 200 yards from the sea. I secured a mortgage and we moved into this nice detached house in 1958, but I was still travelling to London each day by train (Fig. 5.1).

Time passed much more slowly and at the end of the first year I took and passed the Primary Fellowship Examination in detailed

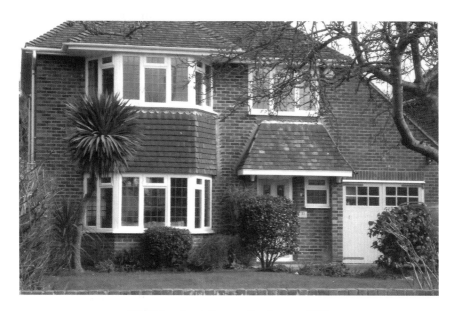

Fig. 5.1. South Steyne, Rustington, 1958.

anatomy, and a modest amount of Physiology and Pathology. Two 2-hour papers in anatomy and a particularly grilling viva by another professor of anatomy.

As the second year wore on, an irritation developed to get back into the clinical field. This highly delighted the Professor who said 'I suppose you will now be itching to get back to the blood and guts of your chosen lifestyle!' Come August there was a vacancy as a Junior Registrar in my old Firm back at the hospital and the Professor finally relented and released me. In October 1958, I returned to the Green Firm now as Junior Registrar.

What did I learn from this period? Firstly, one finished up with a fairly shrewd idea of how the body hung together anatomically — an important stack of knowledge when faced years later with some problem in the operating theatre. Secondly, a further dose of academia and ability to use a library and to write a scientific paper. Thirdly, one developed a modest ability as a teacher of undergraduates.

A useful additional experience during these previous 18 months was that apart from our duties in the Anatomy Department a relationship had been set up between previous demonstrators and a few local General Practitioners. This entailed doing evening surgeries and night calls for the practice, most of which were in the Hackney or Hoxton areas. The arrangement was that at about 6.00 pm the GP departed off to his home in Highgate or Hampstead and we would for a suitable fee take over and do his evening surgery followed by sleeping over night on the premises to take any calls if required.

The GPs were totally pragmatic about all this and when I was first interviewed and approved the doctor instructed me on a few details. The number of patients arriving was usually around 20 persons. 'The first rule is never examine a patient or get them to strip off as they will think you are going to assault them. You can apply your stethoscope to the chest through overcoats etc. — you won't hear anything but they won't know. Look wise and give them some medicine. Look over there!' Behind the curtain surrounding the examination area there was an enormous pile of boxes of drug samples piled high on the examination couch. 'You can usually find something that will impress them! If someone comes in who is obviously ill or damaged, immediately ring Casualty at Barts and say you are sending a patient in. If serious, send for an ambulance to take them. It is no good you trying to do something when they need an X-ray.' In this way, the evening surgery used to be over in about an hour and a half. If you were staying the night there was an old iron bedstead in a corner of the surgery where one could camp down, read and sleep. In the morning a delightful Irish housekeeper would give you a call and serve an enormous breakfast in her sitting room! Sausages, eggs, bacon, tomatoes etc. £6.00 per surgery, plus £10 for a night call. Very useful in those days. Another practice in Croydon was more active and the first night I turned up there at least 25 persons were already waiting. How on earth could one get through this lot — the evening turned out to be a sort of battle of wits to sort out the essentially ill person and for the rest to get a prescription written as soon as possible and get the patient out of the surgery! Not the way to practice good medicine!

In retrospect, in this 18-month period I was very glad I had been exposed to at least some National Health Service General Practice and I became much more sympathetic to a GP's life in general and what seemed their somewhat thankless task at that time.

I have often wondered over the years how can anyone possibly know what this sort of medical practice is about unless they have been actively exposed to it. The administrators and politicians come up with ideas to reform the whole process about every five years. I would suggest they take in a number of GP's surgeries for a month or two and see medicine at the work face before they publish another 200-page report and demonstrate another theoretical solution to these very interesting and chronic problems which were quite apparent in 1957 and now in 2016 are approaching a period of meltdown due to patient numbers and paucity of GP appointments available.

Chapter 6

Junior Surgical Registrar

I returned to the Green Firm as Junior Registrar in October 1958 to Consultants Mr A. W. Badenoch and Mr I. P. Todd. I attended Mr Todd's operating list on a Tuesday, this time dealing mainly in colonic and rectal surgery. Mr Todd was an excellent and meticulous surgeon and I learnt much in surgical technique from him, but unfortunately the type of procedures he undertook were too complex for me to do at this stage and I could do little more than assist, although I now advanced to doing hernias, appendices, excisions of small cutaneous, lesions and at least two simple mastectomies. At last, I was on my surgical way using a scalpel on my own and the relatively minor procedures gave little cause for personal anxiety. Rounds and outpatient clinics filled up the remaining days. Duty days provided more scope for individual activity with the odd appendix, lacerations and fractures to treat again with plaster of Paris splinting. I had to call Mr Todd in for one bleeding gastric ulcer which required a partial gastrectomy, at this point beyond my capabilities.

So the year passed pleasantly. The Senior Registrar was a likeable ex-Naval Surgeon who perhaps regarded our duty day a little light heartedly. He kept a horse at a farm in Steeple Bumpstead in Essex and used to take off quite frequently saying 'Hold the fort old boy, just going to ride the little mare — give me a ring if you get stuck.' (We presumed this was a horse!) He showed me how to do a gut resection on a piece of rubber tubing dividing it and putting it together again with the necessary suturing. 'There you are old boy you are fit to take out a bit of bowel as necessary!' Luckily, I had no need to attempt this at my 'kindergarten stage' but the induced anxiety that something might turn up which I could not cope with was ever present.

My first duty weekend after appointment was memorable in that in the three days in question no less than seven patients presented with symptoms of appendicitis. As I had been advised not to delay in operating when there was doubt as to the cause of the patient's pain, I explored each of them. Five had acutely inflamed appendicitis. Two were indeterminate. The crunch came on the Monday morning round with Mr Badenoch introducing each patient I had operated upon. When we reached number four Mr Badenoch began to look at me a little strangely, 'had he appointed some sort of surgical maniac?' When we got to the patients six and seven, he began to look a little dazed. All the patients did well and I have never again seen so many cases of appendicitis present in such a short time. That's surgery!

Little incidents cropped up such as the evening when a very nice man arrived in Casualty with a note from the Professor of Surgery at Barts and who was also at that time President of the Royal College of Surgeons. The note said "Dear Dr, will you please look after this old and valued member of the College staff who I think has pneumonia" I examined the patient and to my horror concluded he was not suffering from pneumonia but acute appendicitis and patients at this age do not usually suffer from appendicitis! What to do? It is 10.00 pm. Do I ring the Professor at home and tell him of my findings? Clearly, I had to. The Professor was very pleasant and said 'Well Wickham if that's what you think please operate on him and come to my office at 10.00 am tomorrow to tell me what you found!' A scintillating surgical career seemed to be in acute danger of an early crash into the buffers!

I operated with my knees knocking and thank God he had appendicitis. The Professor was *very* interested in the morning! Such small events as this take years off one's life and considerably narrow the coronary arteries — all part of becoming a surgeon! It seemed that this was a system of trying one out without endangering the patient. I think all my chiefs during my training probably sized one up and slackened the leash when they thought it was appropriate. Help was always at hand further up the chain if required. It was I suggest like learning to fly and the day coming when your instructor knowing you were now capable allowed you to go solo.

This appointment enabled me to do an adequate amount of book study and towards the end of the year I was able to sit my final FRCS examination relying upon a satisfactory amount of theoretical knowledge and luck with my clinicals and vivas. Amazingly, I satisfied the examiners and was awarded the coveted letters.

On returning to the hospital, various comments were received. One from Mr Todd 'You don't deserve it you don't know enough surgery.' This was totally accurate! Secondly from another old and wise physician 'That's one of the worst day's work you have ever done. You will from now on only be able to be a surgeon and not a doctor. I hope you are mentally but more importantly physically fit for it.' A very hearty welcome to the world of surgery.

Vignettes from these years

(1) I took two weeks holiday prior to the Fellowship exam and sat at home reading two surgical textbooks cover to cover, one twice! How I did not get deep vein thrombosis I do not know as my mother brought my meals to me sitting in the armchair.

(2) The FRCS examination is engraved on my mind. The written papers were as expected. One question on angiomas (blood

vessel abnormalities), viz. port wine stains etc., I would never have been able to answer if I had not read about it two weeks previously. Phew, complete luck!

The clinical examination was taken in one day at the Examination Halls, Queens Square, Bloomsbury. Long case — a man fortunately for me with multiple angiomas all over his lower abdomen and legs and the angiomas marked out for Deep X-ray Therapy plus multiple hernias. I was flabbergasted. My new found knowledge also got me out of this one! Seeing all the markings ready for radiotherapy gave the game away as to what was the correct treatment which I was able to discuss at length with the Examiner! Secondly, a woman with an apparent bunch of grapes hanging from one breast. 'I don't know Sir, I have never seen anything like this.' 'That's what this exam is about' Draw your own conclusions. In another tight spot. Took a wild guess. 'Cancer Sir, needs a mastectomy.' 'Correct.' Finally, a medical student with a locked knee joint after a game of rugby who had already been examined several times. I placed my hand delicately on the knee and the patient cried out 'I've had enough of this.' The examiner said 'You should be more gentle' — doomed. Hated the medical student.

Finally, the pathology viva at the Royal College of Surgeons — so, so. One good question — what would you do with a patient in clot retention after a prostatectomy? Here I was ahead of the game having worked with Mr Badenoch in Urology. 'Many hard hours on the bladder syringe Sir!' which raised a small laugh.

A bit doubtful as I attended the group session at the bottom of the staircase of the College as the Beadle read out the numbers of successful candidates of the day. Of about 30 candidates three were numbered! I was one! I had made it. 'Will these candidates proceed up the staircase to the Examiners Room to meet them over a glass of sherry?' I was too dazed to remember the details. Suddenly faced with some of the Principal surgeons in the country and the hand being shaken and photos being taken.

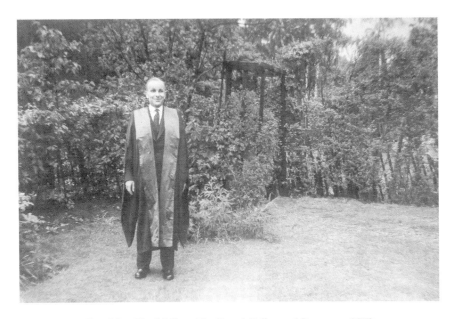

Fig. 6.1. Final fellowship, Royal College of Surgeons, 1959.

'Could you now please sign the Register and your certificate?' My hand was totally disconnected from my nervous system as is demonstrated by the spider scrawl on the document I now have before me! I WAS A SURGEON! Ho! Ho! But a long, long way to go yet. Rang mother. 'This is 'Mr Wickham' speaking. No tears this time (Fig. 6.1)!'

Chapter 7

Middle Grade Surgical Registrar

My appointment was due to finish shortly and I now urgently needed a Middle Grade Registrar appointment to gain more badly needed experience in general surgery. I applied for several jobs. I was turned down at St Thomas's and the Middlesex Hospitals but managed to get a post at The Royal Postgraduate Medical School in Hammersmith Hospital in West London (Fig. 7.1). It is interesting to note in retrospect the various London hospitals which turned me down over the years!

This was a two-year rotating appointment: eight months with Professor Ian Aird, eight months with Mr R. H. Franklin and eight months with Mr R. Shackman. Alongside these commitments were a secondary parallel task — a period of 18 months peripheral vascular surgery with Mr Peter Martin and 6 months cardiac surgery with Mr Cleland and Mr Bentall. This arrangement though busy nicely covered the whole spectrum of General Surgery but the most valuable element of all my training was the peripheral vascular surgery. Mr Martin was an excellent teacher and I was later shown how to and allowed to perform major vascular operations such as aortic resections and other grafting operations. The cardiac experience was very useful but there was no chance of performing any surgery and one worked purely as an assistant.

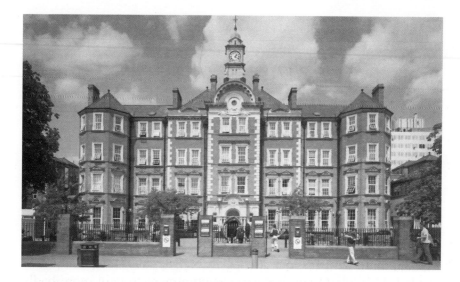

Fig. 7.1.   Hammersmith Royal Postgraduate Hospital, 1960.

Hammersmith Hospital at this time was at the forefront of experimental academic medicine, especially on the medical side with such luminaries as Professor John McMichael in Cardiology and Dr Sheila Sherlock in liver disease. In surgery, Dr Melrose and Dr Dempster were busy with the development of cardiac bypass pumps to allow the patient's own heart to be stopped for open heart surgery etc., all totally stimulating and this was all combined with rounds and clinico-pathological conferences.

Hammersmith at that time was regarded as a somewhat maverick institution by the rest of medical London. On several occasions, I was asked 'What on earth persuaded you to go and work in that mad house!' or words to that effect. On the contrary, it was probably one of the most exciting and important parts of my whole training. There were so many stimulating Surgeons and Physicians and so much experimental clinical work going on that I was totally enveloped in the various progressive academic medical procedures that were being developed. For instance, while working in Mr Shackman's

Department of Urology, I was exposed to the first artificial renal dialysis machine in the UK — the Kolf, developed by Professor Kolf in Holland during the German occupation.

This was also the first department to develop a repeated dialysis regime in the UK and which commenced thanks to the introduction of the arteriovenous vascular shunt. At this time, patients with acute renal failure could sometimes be dialysed once or twice to tide them over in the hope their kidneys might recover function. When I started on the machine, each dialysis required vascular access to major femoral vessels by a full surgical operation. This could obviously only be carried out a very limited number of times. Early in my appointment, Mr Shackman was able to obtain a small silicon rubber shunt directly from Professor Kolf then in Seattle, that could be inserted into the radial artery and vein at the wrist of the patient. The shunt was constructed so that once implanted it could be detached at its centre and one end would remain connected to the artery and one to the vein of the patient. The free ends could then be connected to the machine each time a dialysis was required and then reconnected to re-establish the patient's circulation as often as was necessary to enable multiple treatments to be undertaken. The first patient was a tower crane operative who had fallen to the ground from a great height and was in acute renal failure. He was dialysed about eight or nine times and survived as his kidneys recovered. The dialyser or artificial kidney was a 6-ft horizontally mounted long drum about 3 ft in diameter which rotated in a bath of heated dialysis fluid almost the size of a domestic bathtub. A clear thin plastic tube of about 20 ft in length was wrapped round the rotating drum and the patient's blood was pumped through the tube which continuously dipped into the bath fluid thus allowing dialysis of the blood to take place. The whole procedure taking about six hours needed to be supervised by a doctor as occasionally the tube could rupture and the patient could bleed into the bath fluid. A large red button stopped the procedure if the bath fluid was seen to turn red! Later, of course, the machinery became much simplified, functioned automatically and the whole dialysis bath was finally reduced to the size of a large pedal bin with disposable plastic coils. This was all very exciting as it was a prelude to all chronic repetitive dialysis and to renal transplantation.

With Mr Martin on the vascular side, arterial grafting was just becoming routine with newer graft materials being tried all the time. Graft clotting was, however, a complication. This was thought to be due to the lack of electrical surface charge on the graft lining. Normal blood vessels have a negative electrical charge of approximately minus 40 millivolts on the vessel lining which it was thought prevented the also negatively charged formed particles, the red, white cells and platelets in the blood being deposited and cause a thrombotic obstruction because of the repellent charge that they carried being similar to the surface charge of the vessel wall. Mr Martin contacted the Imperial Chemical Industries (ICI) factory in Cheshire, who were then producing surface charged synthetic materials such as nylon, Teflon etc. which was used for furnishing fabric and particularly curtains which without treatment frequently bunched up due to the electrostatic charges which developed when moved. The company provided us with variously charged nylon, Teflon or other plastic sheets which prevented this effect and grafts made from these materials were much more effective. Mrs Martin machined these sheets into tubes of suitable size on her sewing machine. We had previously had to use her discarded nylon underwear!

I also performed a number of laboratory experiments on the charges exhibited by various tissue membranes using an 'Ussing Chamber'. Here, the test membrane was immersed in a warmed saline solution and when suspended centrally divided the chamber into two. It was then possible to measure the electrical charge caused by the active flux of sodium ions moving across the cells of the membrane from one chamber to another. It was also possible to manipulate this flux using various compounds such as steroids or other chemicals which could speed up or slow the process. Fascinating! I had always wondered why the bladder endothelium or lining prevented a back leak of filtered electrolytes and urea in to the general circulation after excretory passage through the kidney and would have loved to have worked on this problem. This question has I am sure by now been fully answered. I produced my first scientific paper on this subject in the *Journal of Experimental Surgery*. Professor Aird did not regard all this as normal surgical research and was not particularly impressed!

The most valuable portion of my surgical training at Hammersmith by far was this time spent working with Peter Martin. He taught me how to approach major vascular operations such as aortic aneurysmal excision and grafting with confidence. Such was his encouragement that I felt that I could now proceed to very major surgical procedures on my own without constant anxiety and reference to my seniors. As Mr Martin was based at Chelmsford Hospital and only came to Hammersmith on one day per week, I had to cope with a number of vascular emergencies admitted to the hospital on my own. Such events as aortic aneurysmal rupture and iliac arterial obstruction just had to be dealt with as emergencies were usually such that instant action was required.

I was now living in a small apartment at Clapham Common belonging to some distant relative and, getting to the hospital in rush hour was difficult. I had just got home one evening at about 6.30 pm when I was rung by a colleague on emergency duty with the fact that a patient had developed an aortic leak following a lumbar angiogram (an X-ray investigation) earlier in the day. In those days, angiography was performed by direct needle puncture of the aorta or appropriate vessels. 'Please can you get back quickly? What should I do?' I said 'I'm on my way. Open the abdomen and put your thumb on the leak until I get there'. He did just that standing with his thumb over the hole for about 20 minutes until I arrived and dealt with the problem. He later became Chief of the British Army Medical Services and we remained friends for years.

Also at Hammersmith, I learnt to produce a reasonable academic surgical presentation both oral or written which I found invaluable in subsequent years. It was expected that you would produce one or more papers during your incumbency!

Another great hazard was the Friday morning Grand Round and Pathological Conference involving the whole surgical staff of all grades. This entailed usually any luckless Registrar who had had cause to operate on a patient when perhaps all had not gone according to plan. Firstly, he had to explain his clinical management, discuss pathological and clinical outcomes and then give a précis review of the relevant literature. He was first taken apart by his seniors and contemporaries and then grilled by the Professor on his interpretation of the literature which was frequently found lacking, this being the Professor's 'piece de resistance'. This sort of interrogation was also suffered by the other members of the Consultant staff.

At last bruised and bedraggled one escaped to live again. Another secure nail in the coffin of surgical training — but boy did you learn! Such CP conferences had lately emerged from the USA but at that time would have been an anathema at most London teaching hospitals. And this is what made Hammersmith stand out; it was difficult to imagine some of the surgical eminences of the time working in other hospitals being grilled by their contemporaries in public!

My six months in cardiac surgery with Mr Cleland and Mr Bentall was of great interest as the unit was then introducing one of the first bypass pumps for enabling open heart surgery developed by Dr Dempster and Dr Melrose which was the first in the UK. One could only assist at these procedures which at this time suffered from a high mortality.

From Mr R. H. Franklin in General Surgery, I learnt how to do a neat partial gastrectomy which was the norm at that time for the treatment of bleeding peptic ulcers. He could do this operation beautifully in 35 minutes and he was the most dextrous surgeon I met with in my whole surgical training. He operated without a needle holder and used a large handheld 2 inch 'C' shaped 'Colt' needle for every operation and the end result looked like a text book drawing. It was interesting that the criterion of one's surgical ability was at the time 'How many gastrectomies have you done?' Again, I found it a procedure which very much worried me, i.e., sacrificing a large part of a patient's stomach to excise an ulcer and hopefully reduce gastric acid secretion to prevent recurrence. Now thanks to Hydrogen ion block medication, another slain dinosaur is put to rest.

Mr Franklin's dictum on the acute abdominal emergency was 'operate at once, I have never seen trouble come from doing a laparotomy but much trouble from NOT doing one.' Advice I always passed on to my junior colleagues.

From Professor Ian Aird, I learnt how to access the surgical literature and his text book on surgery was a much admired and used Classic at this time. The irony of the situation was that the Professor was technically a rather indifferent performer in the operating theatre.

So all in all, my time at Hammersmith was totally rewarding both clinically and personally. It was the latter, however, which was by far the most important and would ultimately determine much of the future pattern of my life.[a]

I accidentally met a most attractive and unusual lady while in the operating theatre. I was deputed by Mr Martin to undertake an urgent below knee amputation and as the usual theatre was fully occupied I was sent by the Superintendent to the separate Gynaecological unit where a theatre was currently available. Here, I was assisted by a person with beautiful blue eyes showing over the top of an operating mask. Although I could not see her face I was so distracted by her voice that at the end of the procedure, I, on the spot, asked her to join me on a 'pub crawl' in East London one evening. A truly romantic meeting as the leg came off! To my surprise, she agreed and after taking in the Prospect of Whitby, The George in Southwark and Dirty Dick's in Bishopsgate, I was hooked!

---

[a]The Professor's book was "A Companion in Surgical Studies," Edinburgh: E. & S. Livingstone, 1950.

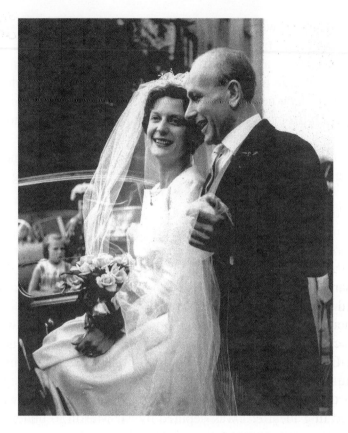

Fig. 7.2.   Wedding to Ann, 1961.

Without the mask she was a winner and remarkably intelligent. Thereafter, we became an item and Ann and I were married in about 18 months. So two very well spent years (Fig. 7.2)!

Chapter 8

Senior Surgical Registrar

Time was again catching up on me and the usual anxiety that it was necessary to look for a further appointment arrived. As I had finally decided upon the neurosurgical pathway, I was preparing applications for a neurosurgical registrarship anywhere I could get in.

Much to my surprise one morning I received a phone call from my ex-Chief at Barts, Ian Todd, to ask if I would be interested in coming back to the Green Firm unit at Barts as Senior Registrar. As at this time the competition for such posts was intense, I agreed instantly. At this point, any further thoughts of a career in neurosurgery evaporated. My training in the principals of surgery at this time enabled me to divert into any branch of practical surgery. Neurosurgery had attracted me by its precision and I thought if I do not pursue my original intent then I could at least attempt to introduce the principals of such delicacy and accuracy into any other branches of surgical activity.

Thus, in January 1962, I returned to Barts to be welcomed back on the Green Firm and a mixture of colorectal surgery and urology. I was by now then far more experienced in General Surgery than when I had left and was much looking forward to developing an interest in one or other of these two specialities and was very lucky to have such excellent teachers as Mr Alec Badenoch, the then Senior Urologist and Mr Todd.

Having had the experience in neurosurgery I was interested in possibly applying this knowledge to the subject of renal surgery. It seemed to me at this time working on the kidney particularly for the removal of small renal stones was a rough-hewn procedure with little attention to subsequent renal function. It could surely be made more precise and less traumatic to the kidney, preserving renal function and save a significant amount of blood loss? This aim then became the subject of my Mastership thesis in surgery at the University of London. I was smugly confident that I was now a clever young surgeon unlike the theoretical tyro who had left two years previously. How wrong can you be? There was still an incredible amount I had to learn but at least I could cope with a number of useful procedures and had faced and surmounted a few stressful incidents. I had resected aortic aneurysms and grafted peripheral arteries and most importantly I was not afraid of coping with a major bleed either arterial or venous. It only takes a week or two to be brought back to earth with some testing event in the theatre to cut one's ego down to size as I often found even after many years 'in the game'.

I worked for both Consultants, more so with Mr Badenoch in Urology and less with Mr Todd although with the emergency surgery on duty day and weekends I had to liaise much more with the latter.

There were numerous operating lists, two with Mr Badenoch, one with Mr Todd and my own list of more minor procedures but it meant that I was in theatre five days a week and every fifth weekend. This was coupled with rounds, being available on call at all times to discuss problems with the Junior Registrar and the house surgeons I found that life suddenly came under a different type of pressure. It was like becoming the manager of a small business.

Getting married had been an added interest! Especially as Ann was now expecting our first child and we were only living in my small bedsit just off Lavender Hill in Clapham known to our friends as "The Hovel"! and we were going to need larger accommodation. On the odd weekend off, we went down to the family house in Sussex where my mother still lived. Salaries in those days were by no means generous and I often wondered whether or not I should have adopted a career in commerce. A number of my school contemporaries had taken such a path and were now earning at least four times more than my rather meagre salary. Occasionally, I was asked to assist by either of my chiefs on evenings and some weekends in their private practices in Harley Street. The recompense for this enabled us to just survive. It had also helped that Ann temporarily become the private ward Sister at the South London Hospital for Women on Clapham Common.

All settled down to a routine for a year and the next step came for me to concentrate and produce a Thesis for the degree of Master of Surgery University of London which was the passport to a Consultant appointment in due course. My attention turned again to the subject of trying to improve and reduce the traumas of renal surgical procedures as currently practiced and especially those of stone disease.

It seemed the sensible approach was to control the renal circulation and avoid the blood loss entailed by incising the renal substance. The next consideration was two-fold, firstly how not to lose function for a short time in an ischaemic kidney and secondly how to preserve function for a more prolonged period to allow a more meticulous approach to the stone removal? Obviously, this was going to entail a considerable amount of investigative research work and how to include this in an already quite packed week was difficult to visualise.

Chapter 9

Fulbright Scholarship USA

Suddenly luck tricked in again. Barts had for several years been in an exchange programme at Senior Registrar level with the University of Denver, USA under the auspices of Professor Ben Eisemann [Fig. 9.1].[a] I was asked if I would like to be the next exchange candidate and have a year's contract with no clinical responsibility to pursue a research project. I grabbed the chance and then began to realise the social implications that heading for the USA plus wife and family entailed. Ann agreed and I said 'yes'. We were not in any way affluent but finances eased a little as I was offered a Fulbright scholarship by the USA government to pay all travel and a few other expenses.

We were preparing to leave for Denver in the autumn of 1963, but three months before the deadline I was contacted by Professor Eisemann to say that he had suddenly been appointed to open and administer the newly built surgical department at the University of Kentucky Hospital, Lexington, KY and would we be prepared to change our plans and go South. We were disappointed but this in fact turned out to be a far superior environment to that of Denver.

---

[a]Professor Ben Eisemann was Professor of Surgery at Denver University of Colorado. He was very concerned with Naval surgery and also held the rank of Surgeon Admiral in the US Navy Reserve. After his time in Lexington, he returned to Denver and became one of the Doyens of American Surgery.

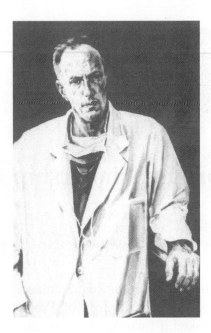

Fig. 9.1.   Professor Ben Eisemann.

It was situated in the 'Blue Grass' horse country which was beautiful with many old deciduous trees and the numerous white railed
meadows of the local horse farms were a chocolate box picture. In
comparison, Denver was rather a desert as we discovered some
years later. The University of Kentucky (Transylvania University)
had been founded in the late eighteenth century as the first advanced
educational establishment west of the Allegheny Mountains and had
many important faculties.

In September 1962, we embarked on the old Queen Mary I and
arrived in New York complete with children, pram and a heap of
domestic equipment etc. We took the train to Lexington, the journey occupying nearly 18 hours with a change in Washington. We
arrived exhausted at 7.00 am and to a temperature of 90°F (32°C)
[Fig. 9.2]. We were scooped up by a delightful couple Jack and
Cathy Gallagher who had been contra-exchangees at Barts the previous year and who remained forever thereafter some of our very
best friends.

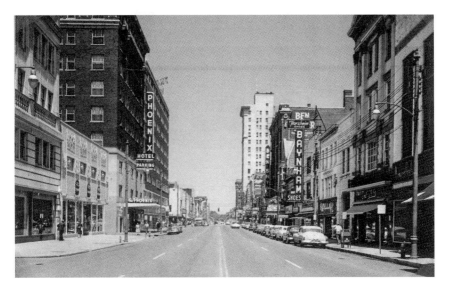

Fig. 9.2. City Centre, Lexington, KY, USA.

They took us into their home, recovered us, and got us established into our own accommodation. We were initially allocated a University flat that was a little basic and small so we looked for our own accommodation and were lucky to find a two bedroomed detached house in a pleasant area belonging to two teachers who were off to Africa for a year on sabbatical. We quickly settled in and I managed to buy an old Buick Sedan 1951 for transport to the hospital and the shops. The Buick was huge, but comfortable with all the equipment not normally available in our cars in England such as electric windows and air conditioning. It was size notable so much so the American friends said 'Gee buddy you a got a big auto there.' Possibly why it was cheap!

So I started another extraordinary year. Professor Eisemann was incredibly helpful and generous, allotting me my own brand new laboratory plus a nice Swedish technician to help and any other facilities I might require bar none. Compared to England at that time it was a scientific sweetshop [Fig. 9.3]. There was an excellent library and facing the entrance on the first shelf there were a range

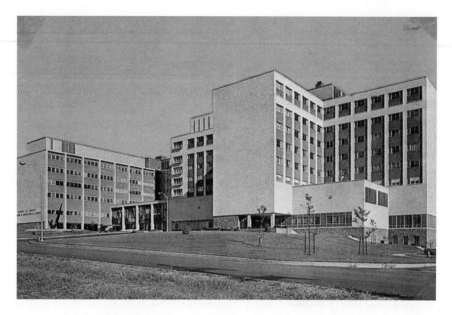

Fig. 9.3.   University Hospital, Lexington, KY, USA.

of volumes which gave me quite a jolt! The St Bartholomew's Hospital reports starting at 1890. Welcome to Lexington!

I settled down to answer the two questions: Firstly, how long can you halt the circulation to a kidney before it loses function? We worked with rabbits as test animals and after a month or so determined accurately that an ischaemic kidney began to lose significant function after 10–15 minutes. Too short a time for a careful operation to be performed. How do you preserve any ischaemic tissue function — you cool it.

What is the then ideal temperature of hypothermia to prevent loss of function? On further experimentation, this ideal temperature turned out to be approximately 20°C (70°F) which would protect the kidney for about three hours. Lower temperatures caused renal damage. Plenty of time to do an accurate procedure.

Thirdly, how do you cool a kidney in a clinical situation? We examined several systems for cooling, intravascular perfusion collecting system irrigation or cold external irrigation. The final cooling method selected was a purely external system which we ultimately developed as this seemed the most clinically satisfactory for practical operative applications. Packing the kidney with ice chips was wet and messy so we designed a system of external cooling coils that could be quickly placed around the kidney and through which various coolants could be circulated such as ice/alcohol or ice water. We could cool the rabbit kidneys to 20 degrees Centigrade very quickly but as we found later it took about 7–10 minutes to cool a human organ to the same temperature. The dry ice/alcohol mixture actually cooled the kidney quickly but easily shot well below the targeted temperature which was not a good idea as the coils froze to the renal surface causing damage so we finally turned to iced water which appeared safer to use and easier to get hold of in an operating theatre environment. I began to write all of this up and it was then almost time to return home.

We had many wonderful times and experiences in Kentucky and the locals both lay persons and medicals were totally pleasant and helpful. We were taken to some beautiful spots — a local Hunt Club was one. The buildings were literally and actually mid-eighteenth century and there was an active Hunt with members dressed in black and scarlet as in the UK! We visited the various horse farms and stables — three English Derby winners at stud!

Another interesting finding was that Lexington was in a non-alcoholic or dry county area. If you needed alcohol, you had to drive to the county line about 5 miles south. Very strange when Kentucky was famed for its Bourbon Whisky. A principal sport was the so-called 'Sulky racing'. Small two wheeled vehicles drawn by highly trained ponies achieving speeds of 30–40 miles per hour. The local venue for this was a large racing stadium called Queensland or 'the Trots'. You sat in a track side first floor glass fronted booth, had supper and watched the racing. Another entertainment there was seeing the especially trained dressage horses taught to walk in five different gaits on command. An amazing sight.

Other attractions were the monthly "cultural events" in the university stadium among which we saw the Berlin Philharmonic Orchestra, The Bolshoi Ballet, South American dance groups and basketball etc. — more 'culture' than I had ever been able to avail myself of in London particularly as the events were free to university staff and families on the University Campus [Fig. 9.4].

One of the Chiefs at the hospital was a marvellous old gentleman in his mid-eighties who was still a practising Urologist. He told great stories of when he started practice in the 1920s patients from the mountainous eastern areas of Kentucky i.e., real 'Hill-Billy' country were brought to Lexington on rafts floated down the Kentucky river because no significant roads existed at that time. He had a beautiful porticoed house in the 'Gone with the Wind' style with sweeping lawns and peacocks strutting around where we were entertained on several occasions. Being English, we were for a time a bit of a novelty.

Various concomitant events occurred while we were in the United States. On 22 November 1963, President Kennedy was assassinated in Texas which caused an enormous reaction in Lexington.

Lexington was slightly to the north of the more ethnically divided adjacent southern states such as Georgia and Tennessee

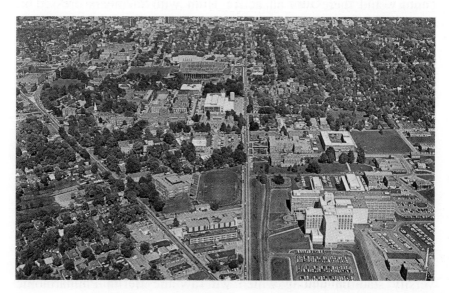

Fig. 9.4.   University Campus, Lexington, KY, USA.

which at that time had quite severe restrictions on the black population. Schools were not integrated and children were bussed daily often over quite long distances to segregated black or white schools. In public transport, black and whites were segregated to specific areas and in trains and some hotels and shops they were likewise divided. Martin Luther King was very active at this time in the States in an attempt to achieve a more liberal environment. Lexington was moderately liberal and we came across no direct unpleasantness.

The assassination of Kennedy produced a very interesting reaction in the hospital at Lexington. In mid-afternoon as the news broke the whole organisation came to a sudden halt, when the attitude of various staff members to the event was alarming. Most staff found the whole episode distressing and a moral disaster, however, a significant proportion of staff were not quite celebrating but were saying this was one of the best things that had happened to this country as it gets rid of a wretched politician. It was this event that changed our own attitude to life in the USA for I had been offered a good personal permanent appointment in Lexington rather than return to England. Our feeling at the time was that we would not be happy in such an ethnically and politically divided society.

The second major event in our stay was that my mother was coming to visit for six weeks holiday and spend Christmas with us. Things turned out far differently. She sailed on the Queen Elizabeth I in about November of 1963. We were going to have a short holiday and arranged to pick her up in New York in the ancient Buick and then come south through Williamsburg and do some sightseeing in Virginia.

Events altered everything. I had dropped the family off en route in Washington and driven up to New York to pick up my mother and expected to be back that day. I arrived at the pier to hear the Tannoy calling for Dr Wickham to come to the office. When I arrived, I was met by my mother in a wheelchair looking totally white having had a severe gastric haemorrhage on the way over.

She was handed over to me and that was that. I managed to phone Ann and asked her to make her way home by train and

I managed to get my mother into the car and began to drive as rapidly as possible to Lexington where I could get some sensible assistance. En route in Pennsylvania my mother vomited more blood and was very poorly. We got nearly as far as Pittsburgh at about 8.00 pm. I felt we should stop, spend the night in a motel and complete the journey in the morning. At about 10.00 pm, she bled again and I felt that she must get into hospital. There was a small hospital in the nearby town and I managed to get her into the car again. In Casualty which was a little basic, a local GP on duty was called in. He took one look at my mother, who was by then a little yellow, and said 'she is in alcoholic liver failure. I will arrange liver function tests in the morning.' He himself had obviously had a little to drink as well. I said 'She has had about three glasses of sherry in her whole life' and he departed. I knew she would have to stay the night and I thought that at least someone would have enough sense to put up even a saline drip and I had to leave her in the care of the nurses. I returned to the motel, could not sleep but telephoned Professor Eisemann at 6.00 am. He said 'she will die up in those hills — just get her to Pittsburgh and I will fix it at that end.' I arranged for a local ambulance which incidentally did double duty as a hearse to come to the hospital for 8.00 am. I returned and informed the staff that my mother was going to Pittsburgh. The nurse in charge said I couldn't take her until the doctor had seen her at 10.00 am. I asked for his telephone number and phoned him. He said 'she can't go 'till I see her'. I put the phone down and said to the nurse that he had said 'ok' and we loaded her into the ambulance for the 100-mile drive to Pittsburgh.

Professor Eisemann had arranged for one of his colleagues, the local GI surgeon Professor Bahnson, to take over. Incidentally, we were delayed outside the hospital in the ambulance while my bank account was checked to make sure I could pay any fees arising (interesting to compare this to the UK and the NHS emergency medical systems). Finally she was admitted, given an immediate transfusion of four units of blood and looked as if she might survive. Four days later, she was stable and was loaded into the car and we made it to Lexington in about six hours. She stayed at home for about a month and gradually recovered but then in the middle of the night she had another bleed. I phoned Professor Eisemann again and he said 'Go to the hospital and get two units of blood we will transfuse her and admit her.' I rushed to the hospital, asked the laboratory for the blood 'no you can't have it as we don't release blood out of the hospital.' To Professor Eisemann again. 'Go to the dog lab, get a drip set and saline and I will meet you at your home.' We set up a drip on a broom handle, gave the saline, she perked up a little and we got her into hospital. Two days later a further bleed, Professor Eisemann said 'I will have to operate on her' which he did excellently and performed a gastric procedure which stopped the haemorrhage. She finally came home after about a week and with Ann's nursing gradually recovered and then had to stay with us to the end of our time in Lexington.

A very interesting introduction to some of the down side of the USA medical care system at the time and the second major reason why we returned to England. We felt that we would rather have English emergency surgery and free UK medical care.

But it had been a wonderful and profitable year. So back to Britain practically broke. My dear aunt, my mother's sister, took us all in for three months while we sorted ourselves out and found a small house in Epsom as the Rustington house had been sold. My bank manager of the time was an angel and gave me a reasonable overdraft and said 'I know you have a good future and I am not at all worried about your financial stability.'

Chapter 10

Resident Surgical Officer, St Paul's Hospital

On return to Barts, I was rapidly back to the previous busy life. I continued to write up my thesis in the evenings in our bedroom with our youngest child crying at full blast in a cot next to my little desk! We were now established in this small house in Epsom which we had just managed to afford and I commuted each day to Barts by train. The thesis was finally finished in 1965. I was granted the degree 'Master of Surgery, London University' MS in 1966.

Again it was time to consider future career moves as I had now been a Senior Registrar for four years. The normal career path in Urology at the time was to serve a period as a Senior Registrar at the St Peter's Postgraduate Urological Hospitals in Covent Garden, London. This was a small group of hospitals comprising in total of about 200 beds — St Peter's, St Paul's, St Philip's and The Shaftesbury Hospitals.

The Consultant medical staff was mostly composed of part time Consultants especially on the predominantly surgical side. The Consultants had major sessional appointments as Urological Surgeons to the various London teaching hospitals. Their sessions spent in the St Peter's Group were in hyper-specialities such as those concerned with prostatic disease, benign and malignant, ure-thral strictures, carcinoma of the bladder etc. Although also carrying out more general urological procedures, this accumulation of talent formed a pool for the salvage and treatment of tertiary referred patients with difficult clinical problems from across southern Britain and teaching sessions were conducted for other Consultant Urologists from across the whole of the UK.

A number of so-called Resident Surgical Officers served as junior staff, usually two in number at each of the groups four small hospitals. These were clinicians of Senior Registrar status, and served at the St Peter's Group for one year departing with the cachet of having worked at St Peter's and the Institute of Urology to take up Consultant positions in the UK and abroad.

Mr Badenoch suggested that I should apply for such a post as a useful addition to my CV and to gain a wider urological experience. I applied and was appointed RSO at St Paul's Hospital in 1967 leaving my post at Barts.

St Paul's[a] was a tiny and rather scruffy hospital in Endell Street, Covent Garden, London having in its past been a hospital for the accommodation of unmarried mothers and also had a large venereal disease facility. It had 50 or so beds some of which were devoted to nephrology with a dialysis unit and two Consultant Nephrologists and junior nephrological staff.

I commenced by working with a Mr J. Semple — on the point of retiring — and Mr Ken Owen, Consultant at St Mary's Hospital, London. A little later, I moved to the team of and Mr Howard Hanley and a second Consultant who shall remain anonymous but who was prone to sink two or three pints of beer at a local pub between an outpatient clinic in the morning and his operating list in the afternoon.

Here, I was to learn many different approaches to various conditions and treatments which were entirely new to me and vastly improved my urological capabilities. Having become acclimatised,

---

[a]Poor old St Paul's Hospital was closed in 1992 — see later, and looked scheduled for demolition but was later reprieved and turned into a rather smart residential club and restaurant. It had been the scene of some of the best work in Surgical Urology that had been performed in the 1970s and 1980s under extremely difficult conditions by many different people.

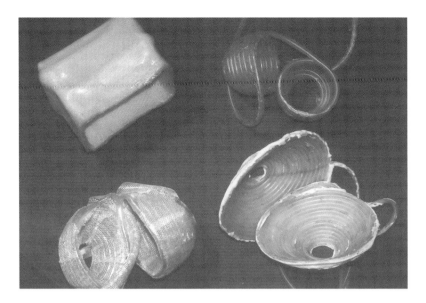

Fig. 10.1.   Experimental renal cooling coils (homemade).

I was able to discuss the possibility of further developing a cooling apparatus for renal stone surgery and explained what I was trying to achieve to both Mr Owen and Mr Hanley. Both were enthusiastic and within a few weeks, I had assembled a suitable apparatus and a little later these surgeons began to utilise the equipment for renal stone surgery. On nights at home when off duty, I made plastic heat exchanger coils by winding and gluing lengths of plastic tubing around cooking dishes or bottles until one satisfactory model was produced [Fig. 10.1]. It worked! A modest number of patients were treated successfully and my first paper on the technique was published in the *British Journal of Urology* in 1967. A small company produced and sold a number of our mechanisms as hypothermia kits over the next few years complete with a telethermometer and disposable plastic heat exchanger. The first experimental Renal Cooling Apparatus and the final commercial coils worked very satisfactorily [Figs. 10.2 and 10.3]. Apart from the stone surgery, I moved on to gain further experience in paediatric urology working with Sir David Innes Williams, who was Senior Urological

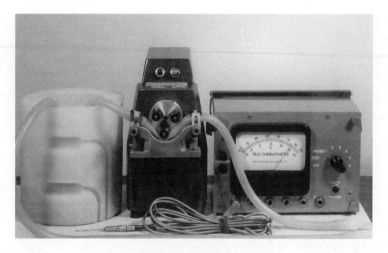

Fig. 10.2. Renal cooling apparatus.

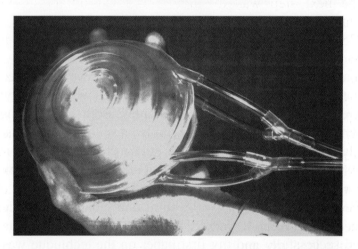

Fig. 10.3. Final design, renal cooling coils.

Consultant at Great Ormond Street Children's Hospital. I was very surprised at the way children survived major surgical procedures that would probably not have worked so well in adult urology as they healed and recovered rapidly.

I found this a splendid environment in which to learn and in which one could speculate and innovate among a group of very stimulating and forward looking senior colleagues. Towards the end of my one year appointment, more anxiety! As usual, it became necessary to apply for further employment. Throughout my career, the anxiety of establishing a continuity of appointments was ever present and hanging over one particularly now being responsible for a wife and family. I was exceptionally lucky in this regard because I was only out of work for two weeks during all the years after my primary qualification. Many more were not so fortunate.

Things moved on and what was to be my future? I felt that I was now a reasonably competent operating general surgeon having had my general training at Barts. My very special vascular experience at Hammersmith Hospital and now coupled with my specialist urological experience at St Peter's was obviously leading me inevitably into Urology.

The next step was to apply for a Consultant Urological appointment, but where? At this time, there were in total about 130 Consultant Urologists in the UK and competition was fierce. Mr Badenoch had hinted to me that the intention at Barts was to set up a new six session Consultant Urologist post at some time. When this was to be was not known. However, in about May 1968, I was informed that this position had been established and was to be advertised. I could only have a go at it. There were several already established Consultant Urologists who were interested, one who showed considerable enthusiasm in such an appointment was already working at one of the premier postgraduate teaching hospitals in London and I was very pessimistic about my chances.

I submitted my application and appeared before the appointments committee. I met Mr Badenoch shortly before the Committee who said 'You know John I have never promised you would get this job.' Hardly encouraging. It was quite an intensive half hour of questioning. To my absolute delight, I was selected! *At last,* I had made it after a training period of 12 years! *At last,* I had made it! I was now a full blown Consultant Urological Surgeon at the age of 39 years and at a London teaching hospital! Shortly afterwards, I was offered three sessions at St Peter's Hospital as a Lecturer at the Institute of

Urology. The attitude of my senior colleagues at St Peter's changed overnight! Life could not get much better!

It did actually as Mr Badenoch asked me if I would like to work some limited private sessions out of his consulting rooms at the London Clinic, 149 Harley Street, which at that time had a long waiting list for accommodation. I jumped at the opportunity. I was by now a so-called fully educated Urological Surgeon who had experience in renal surgery, bladder cystectomy, prostatectomy, urethral reconstruction, etc. I don't think there was much in the urinary tract repertoire that I had not had a go at and felt reasonably competent to cope with, most events, obviously the ego was at full blast! At the same time, I was awarded a Hunterian Professorship and medal of the Royal College of Surgeons for my work with renal hypothermia.

On the personal side, my salary as a Senior Registrar had been slightly more than my new appointments provided, so there was no sudden rags to riches story; I would have to work a little harder!

I did not at this time immediately appreciate the number of situations and events with which I would become involved over the next 30 or so years. Many of these were of my own making, but some appeared out of nowhere and often added significant complexity to my personal and professional life. As Harold Macmillan said, 'one can never be certain of the future. Events, dear boy, events.'

PART II

The Adventures of the Fully Trained Surgeon!

Chapter 11

Consultant Urologist, St Bartholomew's Hospital and St Paul's Hospital, London

I took up my new appointments as a Consultant Urologist in the autumn of 1968 after a complete training programme that had started 18 years previously and having spent 12 years of this period in surgical training. About average for this time, but rather a contrast to the present day training programmes!

Much to my annoyance, the term Urologist especially in the USA referred to the so-called 'Office Urologist'. This was a person who had undergone a basic medical training and had then specialised in what we would call in Europe and the UK a purely outpatient medical type consultation practice doing the occasional cystoscopy or urethral dilatation. These persons were not trained in major surgery and if confronted in the USA with a patient requiring a nephrectomy or cystectomy would then refer them onto a general surgeon. Subsequently, when I was addressed as a Urologist in some of these places, I was regarded as one of those described above. This was irritating and I found talking to colleagues around the world that my twelve years training in most areas of general surgery was far more complete and complex that the average. In fact, even in the UK, a Urologist was occasionally regarded as a person with limited surgical experience compared to a general surgeon. As I was capable of major abdominal surgery such as, colectomy, gastrectomy, and aortic and iliac resection, etc. to say the least this was a little demeaning. Another small ego niggle on the surgical highway!

It is now perhaps the time to quickly review the various stages that I went through in my surgical training in the hope that I can pass on some of my feelings and anxieties at this time. It is a partial attempt to answer the question. How did you become a surgeon? At the expense of some repetition here goes!

Chapter 12

Synopsis of the Various Phases of the Development of My Surgical Competence

Medical Student

At the time of my training as a Medical Student in the early 1950s, there was little opportunity for experiencing any hands on manipulatory procedures. One watched our seniors in the operating theatre, occasionally holding a retractor, but that was it. In the wards, we did not insert intravenous cannulas to set up drips or pass catheters. To my alarmed surprise, we were allowed to pass simple old battery illuminated cystoscopes into the bladders of urological outpatients under local anaesthetic. If a tumour was seen, the patient was put on the waiting list for definitive inpatient treatment. During these procedures because of inexperience considerable urethral trauma was frequently induced and even more so if one was instructed to dilate a recurrent urethral stricture, significant pain was caused and often much blood shed. This I did not enjoy and the patients even less.

In the dental department, one was allowed to perform extractions under general anaesthesia quite often a bloody 'tug of war' and most exciting for both patient and student! Later, one was occasionally allowed to draw blood samples in outpatients and even suture small lacerations.

I can think of little that one experienced that could be classified as embryonic surgical training. My obstetric experiences hardly count but were undeniably 'hands on'!

Neurosurgical House Surgeon

Here, one was rapidly expected to become proficient in a number of practical manoeuvres both diagnostic and therapeutic. I could set up an intravenous drip set and I could draw blood samples. I could perform a slick lumbar puncture, something I found useful at a later date as a medical house physician. I could perform a tracheostomy and pass a urethral catheter.

As far as competence in the operating theatre was concerned, there was little that I could do apart from the occasional skin suture or holding a retractor. All in all not enormous skills, but a sort of feel for mini manipulatory surgical manoeuvres was acquired and a feeling for the ambience of an operating theatre. Also at this time, I formed a nebulous impression that if neurosurgery could be performed so meticulously, it should be possible to extend a similar technique to other areas of Surgery.

Junior Surgical Houseman General Surgery

The first time one views a naked patient on an operating table ready for surgical operation it causes a slight rush of anxiety. Here is a human being which one is going to attack, possibly injure or even put in danger of their life. You are suddenly hit by the enormous responsibility which one is assuming. The best antidote to this modest feeling of panic is to apply the surgical drapes and relegate the problem to a few inches of flesh and reduce the problem to one of a small technical exercise.

Here at last I was to pick up a scalpel and make an incision, stop minor bleeding use coagulation diathermy and clip and tie off a bleeding blood vessel. I gained proficiency in tying a reliable surgical knot and could close a wound in layers using forceps and a needle holder. Slowly a degree of manual dexterity was achieved in using the various instruments learning their descriptions and eponymous names so that one could ask the assisting nurse for the correct tool for the job. I learnt the correct grip for holding scissors and artery forceps and could apply various forms of retractor. One practiced tying Surgical knots using discarded pieces of cat gut on the back rest of any chair that was available.

I think the most important thing that I learnt at this stage was a feel for the various tissues and how to treat them with respect and gentleness. The first time one passes a hand into a live abdomen is a revelation. Here is a squirming warm slippery mass of moving tissue which contracts and releases as one's hand gingerly moves around and bubbling and squeaky sounds are produced. It is quite difficult to take hold of a coil of small bowel without it skidding hither and thither and slipping from one's fingers. It is also warm and slimy. This coupled with bleeding from various sizes of blood vessel can on occasion also be alarming. The liver is quite solid and warm as are the spleen and kidneys. The large arterial vessels, the aorta and iliac vessels can be felt pumping away and the veins are very soft and compressible and all is mobile with ongoing respiratory excursions! The muscular resistance of the abdominal wall is surprisingly strong when one is attempting to hold a wound apart to gain intra-abdominal access and requires significant pharmaceutical relaxation by the anaesthetist. It is here that strong metal retractors may be required either in a hand held by an assistant or self-retaining to maintain a steady opening of the operative cavity.

Quite a lot to take in even before attempting any manoeuvre of one's own. This coupled with your chief's frequent injunctions 'For goodness sake, be gentle'. 'Don't keep moving things, keep steady and don't stick that retractor, forceps or scissors into the tissues as they will bleed' 'Give me some light I can't see a thing' 'Why on earth do you want to be a surgeon you are so ham handed' 'Do try and concentrate on the job in hand and for God's sake pay attention and try and help me!'

All this can be intimidating coupled with the fact that the environment is often warm and one feels very tired after a three to four hour operation as an assistant standing for long periods.

Sudden unexpected haemorrhage can be startling. Arterial blood under considerable pressure goes a long way — often two or three feet across the room. Venous bleeding is treacherous suddenly welling up from a dark recess, and filling large parts of the abdominal cavity quite rapidly so that one has difficulty in finding the originating site of the leak. A lot of blood can be lost very rapidly with a worrying deterioration of the patient's condition. All these episodes are experienced as a junior surgeon, fortunately at the time second hand. The chief is always there taking the load and "The buck stops with you" comes later on. At this stage, one is a protected observer but can see and feel the potential of the situation — 'Oh why couldn't I take up Medicine and prescribe a few pills!' — much more restful but boredom obviously sets in.

Initiation into a complex surgical procedure, I found, can be quite a mental and physical stress. One gets used to it in time, but at any moment disaster can strike and one's adrenaline is always pumping in the background even 20–30 years down the line.

For now, I was enjoying a protected environment.

Junior Surgical Registrar

Now, we are becoming an active part of the work force. One is conducting one's own operating list for the first time and issuing orders and requests to the anaesthetist or the theatre sister. You are at least a sort of Captain of the ship — 'Don't let it go to your head. There are plenty of Elephant traps to fall into.' Important lessons to learn at this point.

(1) Do not alienate the anaesthetists or the theatre sister. They are very much there to help and not infrequently throw you a life line (literally) and drag you out of a hole!

(2) Maintain your composure at all times. Sir William Osler, Professor of Medicine at Oxford University always quoted 'Aequanimitas' i.e. 'equanimity is the essence of the Practice of Medicine no matter the situation'. One never evinces surprise at what a patient says or does nor does one exhibit unnecessary excitement in any situation viz. in contrast to that projected by a television version of surgery.

This dictum is doubly important in the operating theatre. When the going gets really tough, do not panic. A surgeon who gets excited and loses composure gets rapidly into, deeper trouble. The theatre staff begin to fluster, instruments are dropped, voices are raised and persons faint etc., that is, a total shamble ensues. A steady hand and voice at this stage is absolutely essential and the situation usually settles down and all becomes well even if one is quietly becoming incontinent! This knowledge passed down over many years is vital and should be strictly observed.

Now as a Junior Registrar, one wields the primary knife, copes with simple operations like hernias and appendicectomy and at last comes the creeping feeling that you have become a proper surgeon. Do not be fooled you are just crawling out of the crib and beginning to toddle. Cerebromegally can set in at this stage especially as one may have achieved the accolade of the Fellowship of the Royal College of Surgeons of England — this is pure theatrical window dressing — have a care!

Middle Grade Registrar

We are now getting personally mature and assuming more and more surgical responsibility. A good chief will be taking you through more complex procedures and if the opinion is formed that you are not a prototype 'Jack the Ripper', do not have severe astigmatism or have two left hands he may even let you attempt procedures which require a degree of clinical judgement and manual dexterity and on occasion you may even be allowed to go solo. I was very fortunate in this grade to have considerable exposure and instruction in vascular surgery — very essential in any training regime.

This is the danger time for acute complacency to set in. The first two ops on your own may go swimmingly but a pothole is just waiting for you with number three. Now here comes the jolt. The boss is not there and you are suddenly not sure what to do. Here, a small conference with the anaesthetist and theatre sister is valuable and will often provide good advice. They may have taken part in many more operative procedures than you have ever seen! Take it slowly and think. Do not panic and 99% of things will sort themselves out.

Having done your best you should now sit down, have a cup of coffee and watch the patient for an hour and if there has been big trouble phone your boss and confess. Then as I was once told 'You sound nervous, go and have a pint of beer and phone me again in an hour' or something similar and usually all will be well. If you have a good chief, you will *not* be admonished and the patient will do fine. Keep smiling, look big and one day you will be a surgeon!

This aspiring surgeon is quite a normal progression. You are not a dolt but just gaining a little experience as a Junior Surgeon. I know as it happened to me. P.S. If you're in a deep mire, your boss will always turn up and dig you out! Maybe moaning that he has had to interrupt his evening meal. Don't worry he has been all through it at some stage and may be quite amused at your discomfiture!

Senior Registrar

Things now begin to get very serious; you have your own operating lists and are assisted by other junior trainees — not the chief. To gain the appointment, it is assumed that you are now significantly competent. Unfortunately, this is not completely true. You can do fairly major operations satisfactorily, being that there are no unforeseen difficulties.

At the time that I was in this grade, diagnostic imaging had not reached the current degree of sophistication. In consequence, an operation was frequently undertaken with an element of investigative uncertainty. What might appear to be a straight forward tumour removal could turn into a marathon. The tumour could have spread unsuspectingly into adjacent organs with a large associated blood supply that required very careful dissection to avoid significant blood loss. Occasionally, an 'on the spot' decision had to be made that total excision of such a tumour was not possible and probably lethal. When should one back off? A type of decision that your chief had probably made on numerous occasions but you have never faced this problem. Should you press on despite the risks or declare inoperability? Are you funking something your boss would have succeeded in achieving? This sort of dilemma was not uncommon. It was obviously vital to consider the patient's safety and subsequent quality of life rather than one's own reputation. Should you appear bold and competent or rather weak and nervous? Finding the middle way was often difficult. Later discussion with your chief if sympathetic was invaluable. I was extremely lucky in all my mentors.

Two to three years into the appointment I was able to undertake about 80–90% of the usual urological procedures and about 60% of the colo-proctological. This was coupled with all types of emergency admissions on our duty day or weekend. These ranged from reducing fractures to dealing with serious road traffic accidents and I experienced my first DOT (Death on Table) of a woman whose liver was torn into several pieces among many other serious injuries. I was totally unable to put any of her considerable intra-abdominal injuries together and she died of massive blood loss which I could not control. You always wonder if a more experienced surgeon could have saved her but I doubt it. So another surgical landmark is reached and it is not a pleasant experience.

Mistakes were occasionally made, some unavoidable, but others due to inexperience were probably just excusable. Some mistakes should never be made (never events). Luckily, I missed out on this. As time went on, such situations diminished. I would certainly not have wished to have had a shorter period of training. One wonders how many newly elevated young surgeons can fully cope after much shorter periods of exposure.

Finally the Consultant Appointment

The 1970s, as far as I was concerned, had been the most profitable period and one in which I felt my knowledge of urological surgery had been considerably enlarged by the number of renal procedures of various types which I had undertaken. I was now quite confident that I could cope with most situations in urology that I would come across and my appointments as a Consultant necessitated that I performed clinically and surgically to a reasonable standard of

competence particularly by being committed to teaching programmes at undergraduate and postgraduate levels.

At this time, my private practice was beginning to build and it was
very important to give adequate and effective service as people obviously demanded a satisfactory outcome if they were paying directly
for this experience and the buck certainly stopped with one personally. I always regarded private practice as an important part of my
activities because it necessarily kept one up to scratch and blame for
deficiencies could not be passed onto other persons or to the system
as was possible in the NHS. I felt that my training as a surgeon was
now fairly complete and comprehensive. Little did I know what was
to come! This was my situation when I commenced my Consultant
appointments and I hope I have given the reader even a tiny flavour
of what it is like when one steps into the arena of the surgical operating theatre. I guess it is rather like appearing in repertory theatre and
on to a stage for one's first leading performance. The panic wells up
but all those years of standing at the back of the stage announcing that
'Dinner is being served madam' stiffens the sinews!!

What was Then a Typical Day in Theatre
Like as a Barts Consultant in 1978?

8.30 am Arrive at theatre. Into changing room into greens, boots and
cap and mask. Walk into theatre. Good morning to Sister, Registrar
and Houseman and first patient. Answer numerous questions about
ward patients. Anaesthetist pops head round door "All set". Scrub up.
Don operating gown and rubber gloves. Houseman gives a quick
precis of operation to be performed — an open ureteric stone
removal. Check notes with anaesthetist to make sure which side stone
lies. Check side mark on patient and re-examine X-rays. Do not want
to be caught out operating on wrong side. Recheck with Registrar and
Houseman. All in order, patient on table. Clean incision area with
antiseptic and place green towels around and secure. OK everybody?
Sister passes scalpel skin incision made, muscles exposed and
retracted. Peritoneum dissected off posterior musculature, stop bleeding from minor vessels. Look for ureter. Stone is low down so need

to dissect further down into the dark cavern of the pelvis. Can't find the darn thing. Give me more light. Don't want to mistake the vas deferens for the ureter. At last, there it is! Feel with finger, find the stone. Now for goodness sake do not dislodge it up or down or we will be in a difficult stone chase. Gently slide rubber guides under ureter above and below stone to prevent this occurring. 'Knife Sister', gently incise ureter, see stone 'stone forceps Sister'. Stone gently secured and removed. "6 '0' gut Sister." Close the ureter, close the wound in layers with a rubber drain. Dressing applied 25 minutes — dead easy, then into the rest room for coffee. Many more questions from Houseman, Anaesthetist etc. Next op is a difficult one. Takes 2½ hours. Quite stressful. Two small endoscopic cases to do then finished at 12.45. Change up. Quick bite of lunch, if lucky then onto the outpatient clinic at 2.00 pm till 4.00 pm — see about 15 patients, dictate letters to GPs. Hope to leave but Houseman needs you to look at a ward case: 15 minutes. Finished then at 5.30 pm off to Harley Street to review two private patients. This is an easy day with not too much struggle. Home about 7.30 pm, telephone call from Registrar about a case 8.00 pm and tomorrow another similar day at St Paul's with Post Graduate teaching in the pm Still want to be a Surgeon? The pressure continues daily. Add in the occasional lecture day or a demonstration operation either in the UK or abroad and one begins to get a true impression of what this life entails. Busy, but always stimulating! And moves rapidly on.

Chapter 13

The Building of the Department of Urology, St Bartholomew's Hospital and Start of Private Practice

Another year at Barts, all the time gaining more experience and more confidence. I tried to get a prototype of the kidney cooler set up in Barts but for various reasons it was impossible. Now that I was fully committed to a Urological career I rapidly had to face up to a number of unexpected problems. Mr Badenoch had pointed out when I started in 1968 that he would be retiring in about 18 months and that I would soon have to take over the organisation of 'Urology' at Barts. No definitive department existed at that time as Mr Badenoch had been appointed to the staff as a General Surgeon although he had practised exclusively in Urology.

It thus seemed that as the first full Urological appointee, I would probably have to settle down and build an independent urological facility. Until Mr Badenoch left, I worked out of his wards and beds at Barts and all went smoothly. At that time, he had about 35 beds, male and female, for his use.

On the Monday after he had departed, I turned up for work to find that without my knowledge all his beds had been redistributed to the General Surgeons who had been appointed to his previous position and that I had nowhere to practice Urology either in wards, outpatients or operating theatre. I complained and was told that the matter would be resolved at the Committee of Surgeons shortly. I arrived at the committee, made my complaint and was told by the Chairman that 'the Surgeons' had decided that I was too young to head up a department and that consideration was being given to appointing someone more senior from another hospital to allow me to gradually become established! The Chairman had 'one of his colleagues in mind' who incidentally had not been appointed at the committee who selected me.

I was flabbergasted and pointed out to the committee that I was 40 years of age and it was surely obvious that my appointment committee had considered that I was reasonably competent or else I would not have got the job! If at the age of 40 and married with three children I was considered too junior to fulfil the task I would resign at once and seek another appointment where I was more welcome and would certainly not consider serving under a much older person. The attitude changed very rapidly. In the next few days, it was decided by my senior colleagues that I should be generously allowed 8 beds to work out of and one theatre list a week despite the fact that Mr Badenoch had had 35 beds and three lists a week and an outpatient clinic. All this was coupled with the fact that there was still a very large waiting list of patients requiring urological attention. Welcome to Barts! One fellow Consultant had greeted me on my appointment "If I had wanted the job you got you would not be on the staff now." Welcome to medical politics!

This was my first-hand exposure to the attitude of the General Surgeons of this time to the development of an emergent new Speciality within a completely gelled and set in stone hierarchy. And this was in 1970! So, one set to work.

As I had moved up a notch on Mr Badenoch's retirement my previous appointment became vacant and was advertised and I was delegated to be on the Appointments Committee that selected a very good and competent friend, Clive Charlton, to work with me.

Thus, Clive and I settled down to chisel out a new Department of Urology from the granite of 800 years of history! We had no office, we had no secretary, we had a sort of part-time loan of reluctant junior house staff of the general surgical ward to whom our meagre eight beds had been allotted.

It is here that I must acknowledge the considerable help of the hospital administrators at the time as distinct from my medical colleagues. Mr John Goody was Clerk to the Governors of the hospital — he would now be called the CEO of the organisation and always remained sympathetic to our difficulties and we could not have succeeded without his assistance [Fig. 13.1]. He allotted us an office in an old commercial block, 'The Dundee Linoleum Company' in Little Britain opposite the hospital on the fifth floor of a building which was decaying. When it rained, water came through the roof. We managed to employ a secretary, Beryl Beadon, on research monies which I had begun to assemble and she joined into the spirit of the whole adventure. Sitting in the room at her typewriter under an umbrella and with rain water being caught in a number of buckets and basins around her, she valiantly performed her work with only an occasional vernacular expletive!

Clinically, we had to cope with a considerable waiting list and over time gradually managed to acquire a few more beds for ourselves

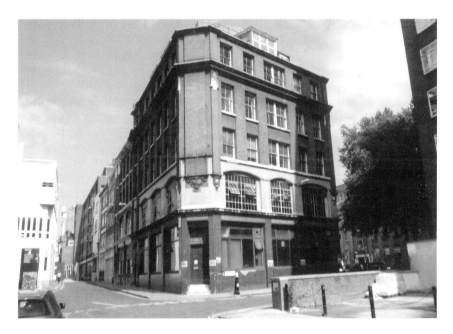

Fig. 13.1. Top floor Dundee Linoleum Co. first office of new Department of Urology, St Barts Hospital.

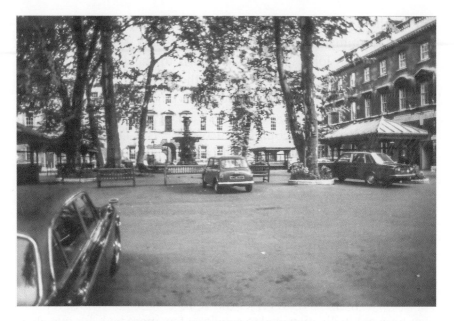

Fig. 13.2. Barts Square, 1977, 7.30 a.m.

by a process of infiltration. We finally obtained our own house surgeon and over the course of about five years we were given a more
respectable office in the basement of the main hospital block, a permanent secretary, registrar and a houseman and access to more in patient
beds. It began to look more like a functional urological department at
last but a political struggle at every step of the way. We started work
very early [Fig. 13.2].

The need to sort out an administrative structure for the department was vital. Firstly, the note keeping and filing system of the
general hospital was inaccurate. After a year, the hospital statistics
indicated that we had processed approximately 25 new cases of
bladder cancer. We knew from our own records that we had treated
more than double that number and it seemed important to establish
a system with more accuracy and we got down to developing a
mechanism for the department. This gradually involved surveying
the whole urological spectrum and reducing it to a record system
that could be easily workable and recordable. Finally, after much

effort by all the staff, we arrived at a mechanism that enabled us to codify Urology into an 80 tick box system as at that time we relied on a punch card system which could contain only this number of slots. This seemed to work quite well despite a few initial groans from the junior members of the department and helped considerably in getting things organised [Figs. 13.3–13.5].

Firstly, we knew exactly what was going on numberwise and we were able to demonstrate that the main hospital registry of clinical notes was nearly 50% incorrect due to miscoding and misfiling. Since then, I have always been suspicious of the numbers quoted by the Department of Health! In fact, the Clerk to the Governors who had been extremely helpful in getting our own stationery printed said to me "That your System and Department stands out as an Island of Sanity in a Sea of Chaos."

Secondly, it helped sort out the problems of unnecessary attendances in outpatients. On the first afternoon that I attended our new outpatient clinic at 2.00 pm, I was faced with a waiting room containing about 40 patients all booked for 2.00 pm to be dealt with by two Registrars and a Consultant. It was obvious that many of these poor people were going to have at least a two-hour tedious wait! It seemed to me that we needed to do two things, firstly, to diminish the numbers of attendees, and secondly, to arrange a timed booking system. I involved the time and motion department of the NHS who came from Headquarters and worked out how long a Consultant or Registrar each took to deal with a new patient or an old patient and codified a group of timed appointments. Adherence to this reduced the ludicrous waiting times for patients and on arriving in the clinic one was greeted by about 4–6 patients rather than 40.

The second problem was how to diminish the number of follow-up appointments, many of which appeared unnecessary. It was here that our new documentary system began to prove its worth. The last box on the whole record sheet was 'coded as Box 80'. Here, the clinician had to record that the patient having completed his or her treatment episode should be discharged or followed up. Many junior doctors were worried that if they discharged a patient they might have made a mistake. It was much easier to suggest that the patient

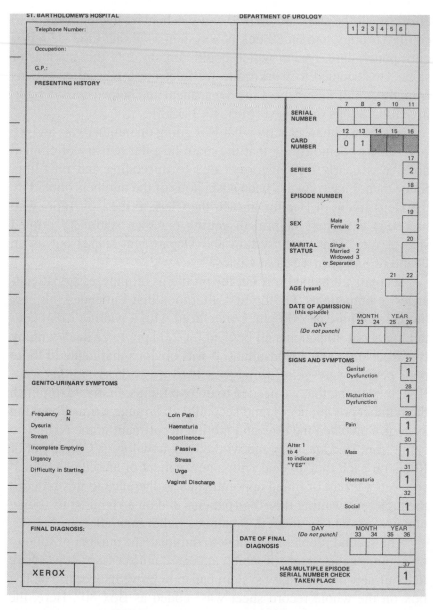

Fig. 13.3. New urological computer system.

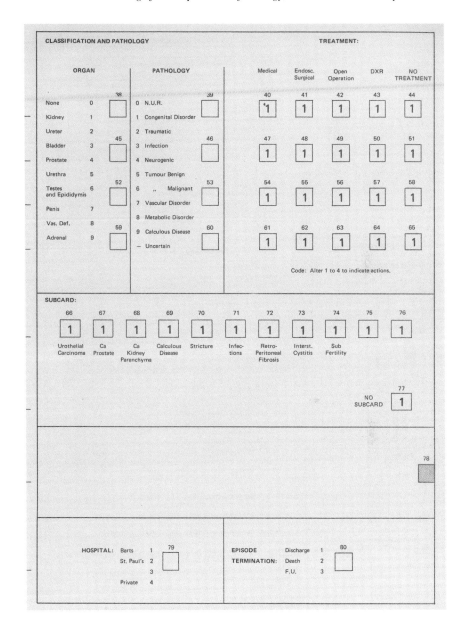

Fig. 13.4. Computer system for the Department of Urology.

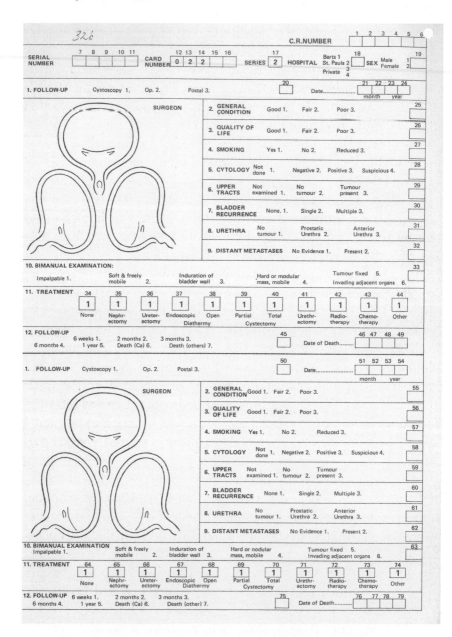

Fig. 13.5.   Final page of new urological computer system.

should come again at a later date for review thus shifting the responsibility of the decision. The only reason for follow-up was now deemed to be either the patient had cancer or had some other condition of considerable interest that we needed to review regularly. All other patients having been treated, the box 80 routine was activated and they were discharged back to the GP with adequate information. To ensure that this system was properly implemented at 8.00 am on a Monday, all the previous weeks' notes usually about 30–40 were reviewed. If box 80 had not been completed, the clinician of whatever grade had to justify to the assembled company why this was so. After a little bit of coercion, this system was implemented and our return outpatient appointments fell by well over 50% thus reducing the crowds in the clinic. We also knew the reasons for follow-up quite accurately. There was an initial problem in transferring the manual box data to our departmental central register and we employed the occasional medical student for a small recompense. A weeks' work of patients took the student about an hour. Luckily, at about this time, the hospital had set up an early computer for administrative uses and I persuaded the head of this unit to adopt our department and enable our data to be recorded on the main frame computer. We had a terminal set up in our office and information could be directly inserted and retrieved — much easier and I believe we were the first clinical department in the hospital to be so computerised.

The Department over five years thus gradually became increasingly efficient. It was also at this time that Clive Charlton who had joined me as the second Consultant Urologist and who had been an invaluable colleague during this initial difficult time had the opportunity of heading up a completely new Urology Department in the City of Bath. After much thought he and his wife decided that life in the West Country and the opportunity to organise and develop an entirely new unit was particularly attractive. He applied for the appointment and was successful. I think at the time many people thought we had had a major disagreement which was certainly not the case and we have always remained very good friends as before and I wished him much luck. His departure left a big gap at Barts but we were lucky enough to be able to appoint another outstanding young Urologist, Bill Hendry, whom I knew well from having being a Senior RSO at St Paul's Hospital.

Bill was totally enthusiastic and rapidly became a distinguished clinician in his own right. His principal interests were Oncology and Infertility, the two areas to which I had previously not given major attention. The congruence in our interests was excellent. Bill was also able to obtain sessions at the Royal Marsden Cancer Hospital and in time became the leading Urological Oncological Surgeon in London. We again worked hard together to make the Barts Department successful. One morning at a BAUS (British Association of Urological Surgeons) annual meeting we presented a whole morning of communications from the Barts Department. As far as I could determine, our clinical results from the various conditions we treated compared favourably with those of other urological departments in the UK and our efforts appeared satisfactory to the managerial organisers at this time.

During this time, I worked on a number of research projects, one being the determination of urethral calibre in bladder outflow obstruction. Together with a Barts Physicist, Malcolm Brown, we devised a successful system which we published. This was so well accepted that it was nominated as the Seminal Research Paper of the decade by Index Medicus International for this work which we called the "Urethral Pressure Profile" and which became widely quoted and used at that time.

I unsuccessfully tried to develop a means of macerating the resected portions of prostatic tissue produced at transurethral resection. The small chunks of prostatic tissue produced were about ½ to 1 cm in size and had the annoying habit of blocking instrumental movement during the operation and at the end of resection needed to be washed out of the bladder often with some difficulty. I conceived the idea that if the prostatic tissue could be macerated to a consistency of a thick gravy like a kitchen blender it could easily be removed as a continual flow device. To achieve this, we carried out a series of experiments in the laboratory using whole excised prostates removed at open operation and macerated them by means of various high speed drills supplied by the Eastman Dental Clinic. We tried various speed drills up to 25,000 RPM at which point the apparatus disintegrated. We managed to avoid personal damage! Unfortunately, the whole plan still did not work as the fibrous nature of the prostate broke down quite well but small fibrous strands of tissue became entangled in the drill and clogged everything. This problem was not solved until the 1990s (see later).

By now, we had managed to extend our bed allocation to a whole male ward of 28 beds and five female beds on another ward. Business was very brisk and in one year according to the hospital records we managed to achieve a 103% bed occupancy! I never quite understood how this was arrived at! We had treated approximately 1500 new patients and dealt with over 3000 outpatient appointments in one year.

Because of our yearly workload, it at last became possible to develop the necessary specialist Urological Ward Services that were required. This thanks for the devotion and interest from our younger Ward Sisters gradually evolved. Successive Sisters were totally helpful in the inauguration of many mechanisms for the improvement of the specialist care of the urological patients. It is hard to enumerate all the improvements that they made but ranged from excellent urinary catheter care to the establishment of proper urinals in the service area of the ward. This last was a badly needed facility for the ambulatory male patients. A clean room was also developed for treatments such as wound dressings and toilet which had previously been carried out with some difficulty on the patients while in bed in the main ward.

This hyper-specialisation was often carried out with difficulty and resistance from the more senior members of the nursing hierarchy but the more correct Urological care of the patients became exemplary and showed the importance of the team approach to the advancement of surgical patient management at ward level. The previous procedures for treating patients directly in the main ward entailed pulling screens around the bed, removal of the bed coverings and then the transport of dressings, instruments, catheters, etc. and disinfectants on a mobile trolley from one part of the ward which often doubled as a surgical preparation area. The nurse then needed to move down to the ward basin, scrub up and don sterile gloves, walk back through the open ward pull back the screen curtains usually by foot or elbow before work could commence. Finally after the procedure, equipment was packed back on the trolley, the patient covered and screens removed. The trolley then passed back through the open ward to the prep area. Very time consuming and not bacteriologically sound.

Now at last at the insistence of our younger Ward Sisters and their persistence often against the more Senior Nursing administration, we had our own fully equipped clean treatment room to which the patient could walk or be conveyed. The door was shut for privacy and cleanliness and the procedure could be carried out with all to hand, gloves, instruments, dressings etc. It amazed me that other ward units did not at that time develop similar facilities. All this required much team work between the medical and nursing staff to promote this. Bill and I established a monthly meeting of Junior Doctors and Senior Nursing Staff in our own homes alternately [Fig. 13.6]. Everyone was invited

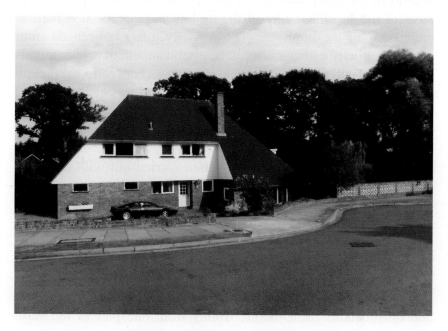

Fig. 13.6.   New house at Esher, Surrey.

to a simple evening supper followed by a two-hour planning session on how we could make the Department function more satisfactorily. Not compulsory, but most people turned up and I think we achieved a number of improvements.

Meanwhile, various intrusions of medical politics which began to emerge filled me with a hearty dislike. I was a doctor and not a sort of a boardroom apparatchik and I must now return to the main narrative of what happened to me as a surgeon.

I was then dealing with general urology at Barts, but at St Paul's my lectureship had been converted to clinical sessions as a Consultant Surgeon and it was here that we were at last able to innovate without the constraints of a restrictive system.

Renal cooling for operative stone disease continued to develop rapidly and we soon built up a large series of patients extending the technique to solitary kidneys and also to the local excision of multiple tumours in one or both kidneys now called nephron sparing surgery. Our interest in preserving renal function was monitored pre- and postop and fully supported by the nephrologists, pathologists and anaesthetists. The radiologists were also most helpful in developing a means of an on table X-ray manoeuvre that enabled us to be sure of complete stone clearance of a kidney at one operation. Vitally important in terms of urinary stone recurrence prevention. Our results were good and we published them in the British and American Journals of Urology and at International Meetings [Fig. 13.7].

A note on my surgical competence at this time deserves a remark or two. As I moved into action at Barts, I felt confident that I was capable of dealing with most surgical procedures that were required of me. But other features immediately hit me.

Firstly, the occasional difficult problem which had not been met before turned up and still caused anxiety although one managed to plod through without inflicting damage to the patient.

The second and much more significant feature was that as I was now head of the department, "the Buck" certainly stopped with me. Until this time, there had always been a friendly senior to appeal to for advice when things became difficult . Now there was no one and I was frequently being put on the spot by my junior colleagues. Memories of the old anatomy demonstratorship returned and one just

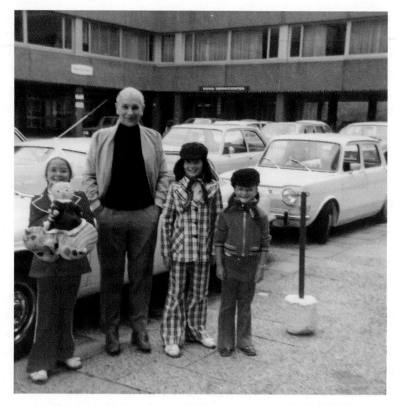

Fig. 13.7. First overseas conference, Amsterdam, with daughters.

had to have an answer and deal with questions arising. This smartened up my attitude to my job considerably. The message was that in any form of surgery one can never relax, sit back in your chair and consider that you know it all. You can never say that you can deal with any situation that turns up. Also, one needs to be in constant communication with colleagues in other specialities whose help may occasionally be critical. Only a fool goes it alone now with ever more complex procedures developing almost daily. There is also a vital need to keep up to speed with new submissions published in the medical literature. The inexorably increasing workload also became a problem. Apart from St Bartholomew's, numerous other events began to intrude upon one's normal activities.

Chapter 14

Ancillary Events:
Regional Renal Hypothermia
and the Intrarenal Society

At about this time due to our Postgraduate publications, I began communicating with other surgeons in Europe who were also developing renal surgical techniques in various ways and established a close liaison with them. It seemed that it would be ideal to convene a small meeting of these Colleagues to discuss our efforts and I wrote to about 25 different persons to see if they would like me to arrange this. In discussion it was suggested that Copenhagen might be a satisfactory venue and we all met there together in 1978. This was one of the most stimulating gatherings I had ever experienced. Over a 48-hour period, we related our personal experiences with this type of conservative renal surgery. Other principal speakers were William Boyce from the USA, Gil Vernet from Spain, Auvert from France, Marberger from Austria, Alken and Eisenberger from Germany, Petterson from Sweden, Rocca Rossetti from Italy, Zing from Switzerland and Gelin from Denmark and a number of other contributors. John Ward, our Barts Senior Registrar of the time, was instrumental in developing many of the arrangements for this and subsequent meetings.

At the conclusion of this meeting, it was decided to perpetuate this grouping under the title of the 'European Society of Intra-Renal

Surgery' and we subsequently met annually under this banner to discuss matters of renal surgical technique with myself as the initial Chairman. Professor Bill Boyce from Winston-Salem in the USA had been invited to our first meeting because of his writing on the subject and although not European became a stalwart in all our doings a tower of information and a most congenial friend. We travelled all over Europe and in 1984 I edited and contributed to a book on our work "Intrarenal Surgery". I found these meetings an enormous stimulus to our work and it was a relief to meet other surgeons who were thinking in ways analogous to one's own and that one was not just a Maverick as had been occasionally implied in the UK [Fig. 14.1].

Over at St Paul's, we continued to develop methods of reducing trauma to patients during these renal procedures. I started by decreasing the size of the required primary entry incisions, finally ending up with a 3-inch vertical posterior lumbotomy wound instead of the conventional 6–8-inch loin incision with much muscular disruption then required to display the kidney. This made the surgery more difficult but produced much less trauma to the abdominal wall musculature and patients were able to mobilise rapidly within 24 hours after the procedure thus avoiding the potential for venous thrombosis

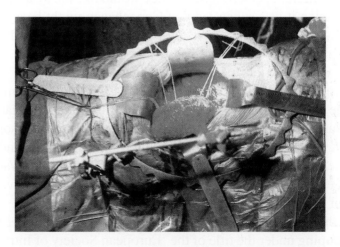

Fig. 14.1. Open renal surgery, St Paul's Hospital, 1977.

in the legs. A colleague called this 'Your mine shaft surgery', but I regarded it as a necessary technical challenge.

We continued to develop the technique of accessing the interior of the kidney collecting system by small radial incisions for clearing stones from the peripheral calyceal part of the system after having removed any large calculi by a direct incision into the major part of the drainage area of the kidney the pelvis [Figs. 14.2 and 14.3].

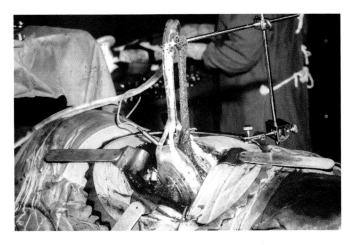

Fig. 14.2. Renal cooling for calculus surgery, 1972.

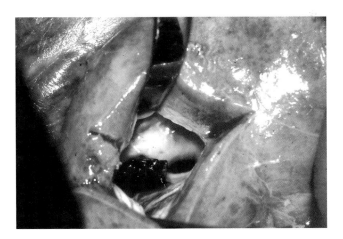

Fig. 14.3. Calculus in renal calyx — kidney cooled and circulation halted.

A brief description of the intrarenal collecting system may be helpful. Once the blood passing through the kidney has been filtered, the resultant urine is collected in a series of passages rather like the branches of a tree. The branches join together to form a major collecting receptacle like a tree trunk, the so-called pelvis of the kidney. It is in these passages that renal stones form and need to be cleared.

We demonstrated that using this method of small radial incisions, we avoided damage to the vasculature inside the kidney and it was possible to prevent transection of the larger elements of the intrarenal arterial and venous system within the kidney parenchyma by careful dissection. The days of the crude bivalving technique were left far behind and we were now producing excellent measured preservation of renal function.

Plastic casts of the intrarenal vasculature were prepared by two of my colleagues at the time. Group-Captain Malcolm Sleight (Consultant Urologist in the Royal Air Force) sadly deceased and John Fitzpatrick who was Senior Lecturer at the Institute of Urology [Fig. 14.4]. I sent John off to the University in Mainz in Germany for three months to Professor Hohenfelner's Department to do functional studies on animal kidneys and to measure any loss of renal function relating to the various techniques of nephrolithotomy

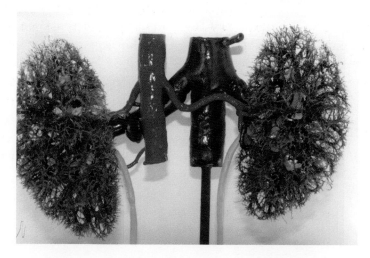

Fig. 14.4.   Cast of intrarenal vessels and collecting system.

being practised at that time. John also produced more casts of the intrarenal vessels showing the damage caused to areas of the kidney previously served by these divided vessels which all helped to confirm the need to protect them to avoid severe functional damage. Professor Hohenfelner generously provided us with all the facilities that were needed and which were unavailable in the UK.

These research efforts were published in our book on Intrarenal Surgery[a] and such techniques enabled us to vastly improve our operating procedures. I also commenced operating on patients who had developed renal tumours in solitary kidneys which left untreated were otherwise lethal. We found it was possible to excise these tumours very carefully, but leaving enough functional tissue behind to support life. As we improved, we operated where there were multiple tumours in both kidneys and in one case removing over seven small tumours in one solitary kidney with good preservation of function and long-term patient survival. This was all very exciting and I felt a little elated that I had at last developed a particular expertise that could make a significant difference to the renal function and more importantly the lives of a number of people.

I also operated on patients with vascular defects in the renal arteries such as aneurysms, these being small dilatations of either the extra- or intrarenal vessels and liable to rupture. As there was time to operate in detail on these problems, it was possible to remove and repair a number of these potentially dangerous lesions, which on rupture could be lethal and had previously been treated by nephrectomy to avoid such a situation. I remember one particular lady with a solitary kidney and four of these aneurysms on different branches of the intrarenal vessels. As I had time, I was able to repair these vessels one by one with the circulation arrested and with subsequent excellent renal function. Another rare but useful procedure was accomplished.

---

[a]Reference "*Intrarenal Surgery*," ISBN 0443 02167-8, Ed. J. Wickham.

Chapter 15

Consultant Urologist, King Edward VII Hospital and the London Clinic, Civilian Consultant to the Royal Air Force

At the beginning of the 1970s, my private practice continued to enlarge and after about five years Mr Badenoch finally retired and I took over full occupancy of the rooms at the London Clinic with my own secretary. Mr Badenoch had also kindly recommended me as his successor on the staff of King Edward VII Hospital for Officers in Beaumont Street and also for the post of Civilian Consultant Urologist to the Royal Air Force which was confirmed. This latter gave me a feeling of considerable satisfaction and a slight step up from my previous incarnation in the Royal Air Force Medical Service, but now with an honorary rank of Air Commodore!

I felt I could never adequately repay Alec Badenoch for his wise teaching and advice. He gave me a full and sensible grounding in Urological Surgery. One of the most important features of his practice was the advice when *NOT* to operate. He fully supported me over some of the most difficult periods of my career with many kindnesses to myself and my family over a 20-year period. He was really the very best Chief one could ever desire and I owe a very large measure of my later Urological Career to his very vital grounding, teaching and very wise advice.

I was glad when I came to retire that I could hand over my remaining private practice to his son David, now a distinguished Urologist, whom I had known since he was about eight years old and handing out the drinks at many of the Firm parties to which we were invited. Also, we were invited as a family to his country house in Wiltshire — equipped with all sports and a swimming pool — on numerous very happy occasions.

At home as we became slightly more affluent we were able to move from our tiny house in Epsom to a reasonably sized residence in Esher, Surrey. This seemed quite a distance from my centre of activity in London, but as the Professor of Surgery at Barts lived even further out I was not particularly worried. Each day I left home at 6.30 am, or earlier, drove to London arriving at Harley Street at 7.00 am when I did my letters, checked on any private patients and got to either Barts or St Paul's by 8.30 am.

By now I had two operating lists at Barts and one at St Paul's each week with an outpatient clinic at both sites. This was accompanied by teaching with undergraduate rounds at Barts and Post Graduate teaching at St Paul's and at the Institute of Urology which occupied some very full days getting home at about 7.00 pm to 8.00 pm. I occasionally saw or operated upon patients privately in my one vacant session on Thursday afternoons or in the early evening between 6.00 pm and 8.00 pm. I began to appreciate the significance of those previous remarks about 'neuronal stress and physical stamina'. Meanwhile, my wife was raising our three daughters Susan, Caroline and Clare and looking after my ageing mother at Esher.

It was now I found my time at St Paul's was the most rewarding. I had very keen, intelligent junior staff and assistants all of whom were as interested as myself in developing innovative procedures to improve our surgical technology. I also spent one day a month doing an operating list at one of the Royal Air Force or other military hospitals such as the Royal Naval Hospital at Haslar in Portstmouth.

As far as my private practice was proceeding, I first became directly involved in medicine outside of the National Health Service.

The private hospitals with which I was particularly concerned were the London Clinic and King Edward VII Hospital for Officers both in Marylebone, London. One was invited to join the Consultant Staff of either hospital if one was approved of by one's reputation.

When I first started in private practice in 1969, I worked principally at the London Clinic then and still now run as a charitable organisation. Namely, all profits were ploughed back to improve the hospital facilities. Ward accommodation was provided by individual rooms most with *en suite* facilities. These were well maintained and there were six floors of about 20–25 bedrooms on each. Each floor had its individual nursing staff under the direction of a Ward Sister. Patient to nurse ratio was high and the day to day nursing care was excellent although not quite so regimented as that at Barts. All wore distinctive uniforms. Most of the nurses were English supplemented by some from Ireland, a few from further afield and the patients had a good standard of care and above all privacy.

The operating theatres were on the seventh floor and were adequate but not equipped to the standard of the teaching hospitals. The anaesthetic equipment appeared somewhat behind the times and the anaesthetists would usually bring their own complete equipment and anaesthetic agents. The surgeons all brought their own instruments prior to each procedure contained in heavy leather cases. The instruments were sterilised by boiling before each operation. Operating suits, gloves, masks and dressings were supplied. There was no intensive recovery centre at this time although one emerged later. The junior staff were non-existent apart from one resident General Physician. Most Consultants employed their assistants from their own hospitals while some provided their own full time practice Sisters. Simple radiology and pathological services were available on site. The principal advantage of this arrangement was that having consulted with the patient in one's own rooms, it was then reasonably quick to get a them investigated, admitted and operated on. The demanding part of the arrangement was that you were directly responsible for the day to day care of the patient requiring at least two daily personal reviews usually first thing in the morning and then in the early evening. One of course could be contacted when urgently required which very occasionally produced conflicting situations with one's NHS work and it was here that the major friction occurred between the NHS and the private sector. NHS Consultants were accused of neglecting their commitments to the health service in preference to their private patients which earned them the reputation of failing to fulfil their NHS contracts. While this might have been true of a minority of consultants, as far as I was aware, all the Consultants that I knew of good status fully attended their hospital patients and spent more extra time and effort in this area than was contractually expected of them. In the NHS, I frequently found myself operating into the early evening and attending meetings well outside the average working day of 9.00 am to 5.00 pm at Barts or St Pauls. I was rarely contacted by the Clinic at inconvenient times as one made sure all was covered as completely as possible and made certain that operations were performed accurately to avoid complications.

In contrast to the London Clinic, King Edward VII Hospital had a more club-like atmosphere. When Mr Badenoch retired, he suggested that I might succeed him at King Edward VII and I was somewhat shy for most of the surgical staff were the senior leaders in London of their various specialities and were a very distinguished assembly. The first time that I admitted a patient and was preparing to operate, I went into the coffee rest room of the operating theatre in a state of tension and embarrassment. I had absolutely no need to have worried. The atmosphere was cordial with many voices of welcome which extended to the whole ambience of the establishment and which was more like a Club.

The rooms were smaller than the Clinic and not *en suite* so patients had to trundle up and down the corridors of the wards on the three floors to visit the bathrooms and WCs if ambulant. Many of the patients were Ex-Serving Officers from the last war and I now talk about the mid-1970s and there was a very relaxed atmosphere. Many patients already knew each other and as they were allowed to stock their bedside lockers with the occasional bottle of alcohol, there were frequently mini parties in various patient rooms which gave the nursing staff a few disciplinary problems. All seemed to get on splendidly and the recovery of some patients was I am sure partly induced by a mild degree of alcoholic analgesia. Incidentally, King Edward VII Hospital was the place to be at Christmas where the whole establishment appeared to be continually humming day and night! This is not a criticism of the situation. Hospital decorum was always well maintained by an experienced team of fierce Ward Sisters who maintained medical normality.

The theatre staff were very competent with the same arrangements as those of the Clinic; bring your own instrumentation which was then prepared for you preoperatively. Anaesthetic arrangements were similar and as one settled into the whole private medical process, one teamed up with one or two anaesthetists to whom one often adhered for many years. In particular, I would mentioned Dr John Samuel, from Moorfields and St Peter's Hospitals with whom I worked in complete harmony and confidence for well over 20 years.

It is notable at this point how much hard work was put in by one's secretary when a patient was to be admitted. First, a room had to be negotiated and booked, theatre time booked, an anaesthetist and assistant booked and finally any necessary blood supplies arranged all to fit in with my limited schedule. Cancelling or moving such an arrangement was a considerable effort, but this problem not infrequently arose especially with foreign patients who seemed to regard ordering an operation as similar to purchasing a new coat or booking a restaurant table!

Most operating at either of the hospitals usually took place as far as I was concerned on a Thursday afternoon which was my one full session away from my NHS commitment although I often had to operate on other days in the early evenings or weekends which made for a very busy timetable.

The major difficulty in dealing with complex problems in private practice was the lack of specialist assistance in the operating theatre and in the nursing care postoperatively. Working at St Paul's in a specialist environment one was assisted by theatre staff skilled in many of the more difficult operative manoeuvres a feature which was lacking in the private sector. The same problem appeared in postoperative ward care where one was accustomed to the specialist skills of the very experienced nursing staff especially the Sisters. It was this deficiency that planted in me the desire to establish a similarly skilled facility in the private sector. This was particularly fired by the success of the Lithotripter and Stone Centre (see later). I made an attempt to approach such a facility at the small Devonshire Hospital also run by the Kuwait Health Office but could not enlist enough support from other Urological colleagues at that time to make the concept viable. It was a very interesting exercise in the psychology of one's colleagues who initially supported the concept then failed to follow it through with the promised admission of their patients — another of life's hard lessons!

At around this time, another facet of the Urological process rapidly emerged, namely renal transplantation.

Chapter 16

Dialysis and Renal Transplantation

At this stage, I was asked by my nephrological colleagues at St Paul's, Drs Joekes and Harrison to undertake the vascular surgery needed by patients requiring repetitive haemodialysis. This consisted of developing small arteriovenous fistulous connections in the wrist or forearm of the patient that would provide intravascular access to the circulation for repetitive chronic dialysis in a similar fashion to the plastic shunts that had been used in Hammersmith Hospital some years previously. I was very happy to take this on having had my previous vascular training and it was a rest from urological operating.

Secondly, the nephrologists at both hospitals were gearing up to start renal transplantation programmes.

First, there was the problem of accommodation for the transplant patients. In early days, it was considered necessary to place the patients in isolation in a single room because being immunosuppressed they were thought to be in danger of infection if treated in a communal ward. Barts was lacking in easily available single rooms, but it was suggested that one of the small single ward side rooms could be used. The patients would require special nursing and if isolated the senior nursing administrator required the appointment of six extra nurses to accommodate round the clock attention, time off and holidays, etc. and the project became stalled. In contrast, at St Paul's two single rooms could be made available in one of the wards and the nursing administration indicated that they could manage with current levels of expert staff and be ready to go.

One summer evening, a suitable patient and donor kidney presented to my nephrological colleague at Barts, Dr L. R. Baker, but we were unable to operate because of the above difficulties so I suggested the patient could be transferred to St Paul's where I performed the first transplant operation in both groups in June 1973. Luckily, all went well and over time there gradually appeared no need for nursing patients in isolation as we had negligible problems with infection. This particular manoeuvre encouraged Barts to come up to speed and rethink its nursing requirements and I was soon doing renal transplantation at both hospitals [Fig. 16.1]. I did not realise what a burden I was assuming! At this stage,

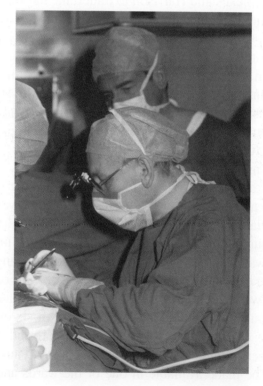

Fig. 16.1. Renal transplantation, St Paul's Hospital, 1978.

preservation methods suitable for kidneys awaiting grafting had not been developed and we had to rapidly accept donor kidneys from patients dying in Intensive Care Units and other sources and occasionally from accidental deaths. From the cease of the donor circulation to getting the kidney re-perfused was a critical period of no more than 3 hours often occurring at night or weekends and calls to operate at inconvenient times resulted in lack of sleep and interference with daily schedules and was becoming a problem. To help alleviate this difficulty, we set up a renal preservation programme at Barts run by a designated research Registrar who investigated both the techniques of cold or warm perfusion to preserve the grafts for a more prolonged period [Fig. 16.2].

Clinically we started using the existing Swedish Gambro-warm perfusion apparatus and our research Registrar travelled around Europe under the auspices of an organisation called Euro Transplant collecting suitable kidneys offered by various units, put them on the apparatus and brought them back to London for transplantation.

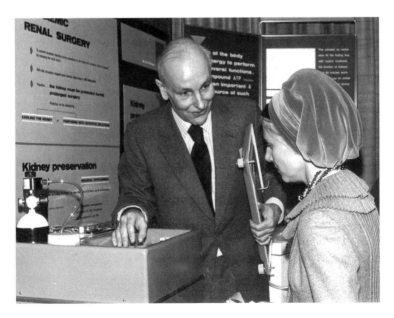

Fig. 16.2.　Demonstrating kidney preservation machine to Royal Patron.

Likewise, we exchanged suitable kidneys with the continent. Much to our surprise, the various airlines generously carried the kidneys gratis and seemed quite happy to transport these mysterious machines with wires, dials and gas cylinders making very odd clicking and whirring sounds. No one ever queried all this! The days of bombs and terrorists had yet to emerge from the less civilised areas of the world. This system achieved nearly a 24-hour preservation period and reduced the need for emergency transplantation at very inconvenient times such as 12.00 pm on Christmas Day! Our own efforts at renal preservation in the laboratory using a warm perfusion apparatus became successful, but too complex for mobile use and when a publication of the results from a worker in the USA demonstrated that using cooling with a specially designed perfusate showed equally good results with a much less complicated means of preservation we turned over to this method which saved much money and effort. We could now simply preserve kidneys for up to 24 hours without loss of function.

Ultimately, the pressure of the transplant programme became considerable and the operation itself which was quite simple had become rather repetitive and boring. By this time, over about a four-year period I was assured by my nephrological colleagues that I had carried out well over 150 operations, mostly functionally successful.

At last, a definitive transplant surgeon was appointed to the region to take on the work both at Barts, St Paul's and the London Hospital and I was very happy to pass the baton and turn to other more technically interesting procedures.

Chapter 17

Disaster: Acute Pancreatitis

All was going quite nicely until the summer of 1976 when one Sunday morning on leaving church with the family I was suddenly seized with abdominal pains. Our GP was called who gave me one dose of analgesics which did little to ease the pain and then gave a second injection which rendered me unconscious and I lost interest in the whole procedure! My wife rushed around and organised for me to be transferred to Barts where I was seen by my old chief Ian Todd, who performed an immediate laparotomy which showed I was suffering from acute pancreatitis a fairly lethal condition. This was caused by a gall stone which had moved into and obstructed my bile duct and caused a reflux of the bile into my pancreas inducing it to rupture. I was closed up and over the course of two weeks I gradually recovered despite a dehiscence or breakdown of my wound which required a return to the theatre to be re-sutured. Interestingly, I diagnosed my own wound breakdown at about 5.00 am but it took until about 11.00 am before I could persuade the nursing staff that there was a problem! Incidentally, the first meal that I was offered after a week on intravenous (IV) fluids was Irish stew! So even in Barts in 1976 the system of nursing was showing evidence of strain as the Salmon nursing structure was beginning to kick in. As an interested patient, I noticed quite a number of incidents which would never have occurred in the 1950s. Very often, the ward was left in charge of staff nurse with no evidence of a Sister or Deputy. There were certainly no complete and regular rounds as in the old days. Frequently, my IV drip would run through and I had to turn it off myself and inform the nursing staff. I was nursed in the open ward with the patient in the next bed obviously becoming intestinally obstructed which took over 48 hours to be recognised and remedied. It was very difficult not to interfere!

After about two weeks, I finally got home feeling extremely unwell, had another attack of pain when I would guess that the gall stone apparently passed on and over the course of 6–8 weeks I gradually got better thanks to the excellent care and attention of my dear wife. It was also the heat wave summer of 1976 and I remember just sitting in the shade of a willow tree in our garden and incapable of doing any activity.

I gently returned to work at the end of 1976 and was doing an outpatient clinic when one of my medical colleagues came rushing in with the X-rays of my gall bladder which had been performed as a check-up. 'You have multiple small gall stones in your gall bladder, any of which could move and block you again, you are going to have to have your gall bladder removed tomorrow morning. It's all booked and Ian Todd will do it at King Edward VII Hospital.' I protested that I had only just recovered but he was quite adamant and I duly had my gall bladder removed and recovered. I was not offered Irish stew postoperatively in this hospital. I returned to work about a month later and had no subsequent problems.

To have a life threatening drama such as this very much sharpened my appreciation of what the average patient has to endure. I was treated in the open ward at Barts and the noise and constant activity was quite unnerving. Also, the lack of continuity in the medical staff with very frequent changes of housemen and registrars was not reassuring. For three days, I was not able to find out the cause of my problem as no-one would pause to discuss it with me. It was only when one of my physician colleagues came by to say hello that I was told of the diagnosis, Ian Todd having gone abroad for two weeks after operating on me and the Senior Registrar being absent apparently looking for Consultant appointments. Thereafter, I was considerably more conscious of a patient's feelings and anxieties.

This reinforced my intention to make sure as far as possible that continuity of attention from the same medical staff should be a priority in my personal practice — now sadly missing from the NHS due to unrelenting bureaucratic interference in the medical process. I had completely recovered in about two months and was back in full activity apart from quite a large incisional hernia which I kept for the rest of my life as I was not quite sure what any surgeon was going to find when he began an exploratory repair job! Unsightly, but no functional trouble!

Chapter 18

Personal Life in the 1980s and Stowe Maries, Westcott, Surrey

As we became more affluent, we decided to move from our house in Esher which was small for the expanding activities of three teenage daughters, particularly as the open fields that we looked out on to were about to undergo development into a new housing estate which was another incentive.

At about this time, our daughters who were in their teens were caught up in the fashionable pursuit of riding and against my better judgement I was persuaded to buy a horse. Ann had been riding a lot in Ireland in her late teens and was supportive of the girls' desire! So naturally 'Spotty' soon became a member of the family but had to be kept at a livery stable nearby. He was an Appaloosian breed of pony white with black spots and of the type that frequently appeared in circuses. He lived up to his pedigree! Difficult to control and quite a joker being kept in a livery stable at some expense!

Early morning breakfast "Daddy wouldn't it be nice if Spotty had his own field to live in?" — the pressure was obviously on and so the search for a new house began in earnest. We looked at numerous houses and one in the village of Westcott near Dorking in Surrey was attractive and appealed.

Meanwhile, my mother became ill and died at home at the age of 84.

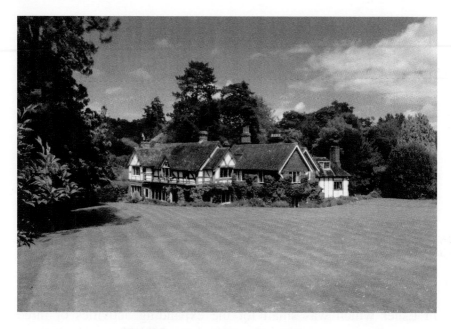

Fig. 18.1.   Stowe Maries, Wescott, Surrey.

A year later in an Estate Agents display we saw the same house. I said to the agent "I suppose that's left over from last year", "No it's now back on the market at a reduced price". We bid again, got the house and moved in August 1980. The house was called 'Stowe Maries' or 'Mary's House' and dated from the 1540s with a number of later additions plus the vital field for 'Spotty' to enjoy [Fig. 18.1]. The journey into London was slightly longer but the house was an ideal background for many happy a family gatherings especially at Christmas when fully decked. Also, our three daughters were ultimately married and had their wedding receptions at home. My journey took me 45 minutes to get in in the morning, leaving at 6.00 am to avoid the traffic. There we stayed for the next 30 years enjoying many happy experiences and occasional sad ones [Fig. 18.2].

My interest in sporting activities in general apart from a little tennis, was and is still absolutely zero but we were lucky enough to have an open air swimming pool which came with the house and which the children and many neighbours very much enjoyed.

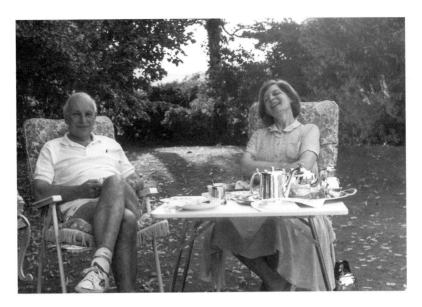

Fig. 18.2.   Tea on the lawn, 1985.

Maintenance was significant and I calculated that with the interference of the weather and repairs etc. each personal swim would have cost me enough to support a complete Olympic team in some comfort.

Another feature of our existence was 'The Donkeys'. My wife, a great animal lover, had always been fond of donkeys and wished profoundly that we should adopt one as we had the field space now available. So one Saturday morning we went to a nearby Donkey Sanctuary and said we would like to have a donkey. The immediate reply was 'you can't have one, on its own it will pine.' Result: two rescue donkeys, Mabel and Lucy were quickly transported to the fields opposite the house. An old stable was restored for them and they then embarked on a life of complete donkey luxury, became the general village pets, visited by children to and from school and mothers with babies in pushchairs and were fed with various eatables, the nature of which we could only guess. Anyway, they thrived doing nothing but eating and standing about and my wife looked after them as part of the family. Speciality early morning carrots. Both of these animals survived for nearly 30 years, one dying just before we moved. What to do with the remaining one? Luckily, the new purchaser of the house volunteered to take over her care and arranged for a new companion for her. She finally died a year later in the only field that she had ever known from the time she arrived with us as not much more than a foal. We were very pleased to have given them what appeared to be a happy donkey life.

Our other livestock was of course dogs. We had had Jack Russell terriers for some years and we still do. These were supported on several occasions with Golden Retrievers, the two breeds always becoming great friends and a constant delight to have around. Quite the little zoo. Incidentally, Spotty soon became side-lined and left us to go hunting in Lincolnshire as the boyfriends moved in!

Another important feature of Stowe Maries was that it was an excellent backdrop for assembling various social functions. It was a very beamed old house dating from 1540 with 'add ons' over the centuries — in, Victorian, Geogian and 1930s style.

I had always been most impressed with the generous parties that had been organised by my ex-Chief and his wife, Mr and Mrs Badenoch. Twice a year at Christmas and in the summer, they would host parties for all the 'Firm'. This included all the junior medical staff, sisters, nurses, theatre staff, nurses and technicians, the cleaning and secretarial staff again often with wives and children.

Ann and I had very pleasant memories of these gatherings and resolved to perpetuate them with the new Department of Urology. Stowe Maries was an ideal venue but had the disadvantage of being about 20 miles away from the hospital and some guests had no personal transport.

We started our own parties on an annual basis in the summer months but always felt it was rather a task for people to make quite a long journey for a few glasses of wine and buffet supper.

In an attempt to make the journey worthwhile, we decided to make the parties more interesting by having a historical theme included which gave any ladies the added incentive to dress up, and in this they appeared successful.

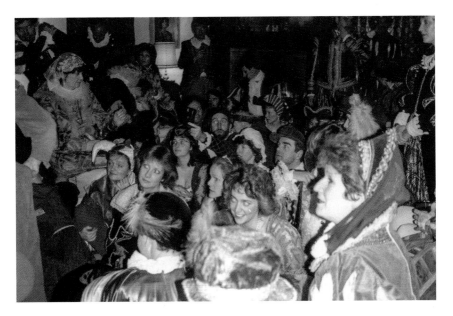

Fig. 18.3. Party (Tudor), 1987.

With Stowe Maries having a Tudor background it was decided that the first party should have an Elizabethan theme. It was rather doubtful if people would accept this suggestion but to our surprise everyone seemed to consider this a good idea — especially the ladies. The result was amazing mini buses were hired and everyone turned up in some sort of elaborate dress [Fig. 18.3]. The food as far as we could make it was authentic and with an appropriate musical accompaniment. The whole idea seemed to be so well appreciated that requests for similar functions then occurred annually so that Victorian, Edwardian and 1920s gatherings took place.

The part my wife played in all the arrangement for these parties was indefatigable and they would never have succeeded without her considerable input. The costumes that the guests turned up in were unbelievable!

Other family matters of course transpired. As we had ample accommodation, we were able to accommodate and look after an old aunt of mine who came to live and die at home and subsequently Ann's mother also came to live with us and finally died peacefully at home. Three daughters had successions of friends to stay so the house was well used.

When I was working in London and latterly around the world Ann had pursued her own interest in the History of Art doing an Open University Bachelor's degree and Chairing the Local Decorative and Fine Arts Society. She had been a founder member and second Chairman of the Esher Society before we moved to Westcott. She was particularly concerned with Church Recording i.e. a project by local NADFAS (National Association of Decorative and Fine Art Societies) societies all over the country to form into groups and examine in detail their local churches and their contents. They then recorded in detail their findings for posterity passing completed accounts of their work to the diocese and to the national archive. Early on she became the National organiser for this activity and when we moved to Westcott she said that she had done enough and would retire. We had been at Stowe Maries for about 30 minutes when a local lady called and said 'We want to start an NADFAS society in Dorking, we heard that you knew about such things — will you advise us how to do this?' Result culminating later in the Chairmanship of Dorking NADFAS, the schooling of many successor Chairpersons and then President for 10 years. To fill in any spare time, she also pursued her interest in antique silver, particularly of the Ecclesiastical type which resulted in her being asked to set up a new Diocesan Treasury in Guildford Cathedral. This she did very successfully and remained Curator and improver of the collection for the next 20 years. All of this was currently running alongside her active membership of the League of Friends of St Bartholomew's Hospital becoming twice Chairman and finally President for an undetermined term, a post that she still fulfils. For relaxation, she catalogued the silver collections of the Company of Barber Surgeon's and the Royal Yacht Club. Activities for which she was awarded with her election as an Honorary Freeman of the aforementioned company and also later becoming Chairperson of the Barbers Historical Society but had no recognition from the Yacht Club! Phew! My daughters 'activities' were another facet of this whole shifting scenario! I hope this may give just a little flavour of the married life of one surgeon in the 1980s and 1990s. How typical one can never know. I was seldom asked to return to London in an emergency once home but such an event possibly occurred around three to four times a year after hours. Excluding annual leave, I was constantly available on the telephone to talk to and advise junior staff and patients. My contract was open ended 'To attend to the welfare of the patients of St Bartholomew's Hospital under your care' except during the period of six weeks of annual leave, and be available twenty four hours a day, seven days a week — a little difficult to do with today's contractual arrangements. Incidentally, I never managed to have more than two weeks continuous holiday. Most holiday periods were taken up by attendance at various International Urological meetings. A similar contract was offered at St Paul's and of course private practice demanded even further personal attendance with rounds on Saturdays and Sundays as required. These were the normal conditions of employment in the 1960s and 1970s. Once a patient had consulted, then one was professionally committed 24/7 with their welfare. A rather different attitude as is currently displayed in the NHS

Other Activities

Alongside all this above, I ultimately became the Editor of the *Journal of Minimally Invasive Therapy*, organiser of various society meetings, National and International. President of the Urological Section of the Royal Society of Medicine, Chairman of the Instrument Committee of the British Association of Urological Surgeons, membership of a number of committees concerned with hospital and operating room design for the NHS. At one time, I seemed to have acquired the services of an array of secretaries — two at Barts, one at St Paul's, one at the Institute of Urology and two in Harley Street. I found driving in and out of London the most peaceful time of the day — no one could get at you too easily and I could actually think and there were no mobile phones!

Slowly, another occupation developed. I had always been interested in cars and over the years had tried several different makes.

The favourite had been a Daimler/Jaguar which I had driven to many places in Europe and the UK and have never been able to part with it. One of our instrument representatives was a keen member of the Daimler Owners Club and encouraged me to join and become interested in salvaging old cars of this marque. In this way with the help of a keen son-in-law Paul, I became involved with old car restoration. On Saturdays, we began to work in an old stable and slowly built up a collection of Daimlers. The trouble with this hobby is that once you have restored an old car one cannot part with it. It is like discarding one of your children and a collection develops. Fortunately, we had some old stables to store them in until we downsized and had to sell. The fruits of our labours are shown in the photographs [Figs. 18.4 and 18.5]. One other problem with old cars is that when returned to normality they still perform like old cars and

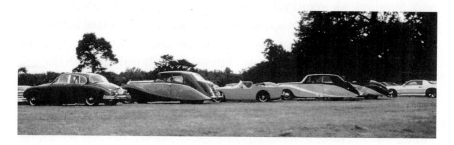

Fig. 18.4. Restored Daimlers.

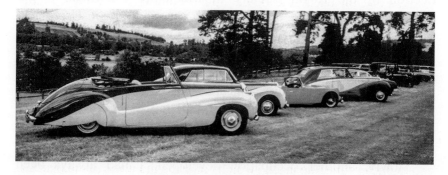

Fig. 18.5. Restored Daimlers.

are really not suitable for use on modern roads. They therefore stand around like garden ornaments and are not used but still require a degree of maintenance. It is not like stamp collecting!

The message that I would leave one with is that should you desire a quiet life, do not take up Surgery. It's not possible, the adrenaline level is consistently high both in work and play. Go into medical politics as a Physician it will keep you active in a more relaxed mode.

To return to the clinical story.

I was still pursuing as *my Primary Object in my own surgical performance the reduction as far as possible of the degree of iatrogenic damage produced in any operation.*

I had for a number of years been consistently, dismayed at the crude and damaging procedures that were being carried out in some specialities. Urology was by no means the worst example of these in its performance but it in no sense compared to the meticulous manner in which neurosurgical and ophthalmic surgery was carried out so why could we not do the same? Is it because iatrogenic damage to the brain or eye is so immediately obvious that enormous care in such surgery is taken? Because the poor old kidney was in general a mute, uncomplaining but nonetheless vital organ that it should receive no less care and delicacy in handling seemed to be quite irrational. A further quick lesson in renal Physiology and Anatomy may be helpful in explaining some of the operative manoeuvres that we were using and developed at this time. The normal patient is equipped with two kidneys one on each side of the spinal column at the back of the abdominal cavity. These are kept in place by a thick layer of fat — known in culinary circles as suet. Each kidney is fed by an artery and the blood is filtered in a mass of tubes in each kidney to remove unwanted waste by the formation of the urine and the cleaned blood is then returned to the circulation by the renal vein. The urine is collected by a series of tubes which are arranged like the branches of a tree with the smaller branches finally joining to form a tree trunk like tube (the pelvis of the kidney). From here, the urine drains by a 3–4-mm diameter tube, the ureter, which conducts the urine to the bladder. Here, it collects and is from time to time voided when convenient.

One of our major interests as Urologists was to free these larger tubes from stones which form in some patients and cause considerable pain (renal colic). The main trouble in accessing these tubes is that they are closely surrounded by multiple small arteries and veins which bleed very easily if damaged. Our principal efforts at this time were to find ways of accessing these collecting tubes without causing damage to all the small blood vessels surrounding them when performing open surgical operations. Then in 1979 life suddenly changed forever!

Chapter 19

The Percutaneous Nephrolithotomy and the Endourology Society and Courses at the Institute of Urology

It was in the autumn of 1979 that my colleague in Radiology at St Paul's, Dr Michael Kellett [Fig. 19.1], had been refining a method of relieving the problem of outflow obstruction in kidneys that had been produced by various diseases. The technique involved making a direct long needle puncture percutaneously into the dilated and obstructed collecting system within the kidney under purely radiological control and then over a guide wire inserting a fine drainage tube. Quite a difficult manoeuvre as the kidney normally lies about 3.0 cm from the skin and surface. The relevant target area in the renal collecting system was sometimes as little as 5–10 mm in size. I had watched this operation developing with considerable interest.

In November, I was presented with a typical case of a 1.0-cm stone in the lower calyx of the collecting system of the patient's left kidney which was otherwise completely healthy as was the patient.

I was due to perform a conventional open surgical stone removal the following day. It suddenly occurred to me that if Michael could put a tube into the correct part of the kidney it might be possible to make the track a little wider, wide enough in fact for me to pass an ordinary bladder cystoscope into the kidney. If I followed this up

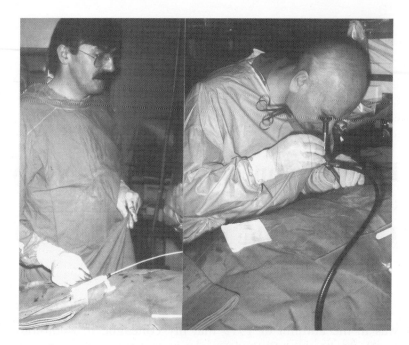

Fig. 19.1. Dr Michael Kellett, Consultant Radiologist on left.

with a small wire stone basket as used for extracting stones from the ureter, I might just be able to see, secure the stone and effect its removal without the need for a major procedure.

I discussed this with Michael and he thought it might be feasible to dilate the track to about 1.0 cm but that this might produce a significant degree of bleeding from the kidney tissue that could produce problems with internal haemorrhage thus making visualisation impossible. On further thought, he suggested that after dilating the track it might be possible to pass a slightly larger tube and leave it *in situ* to tamponade any bleeding vessels and which if left for 24–48 hours would allow clotting to occur and then enable me to pass an endoscope with a decent prospect of seeing what I was doing.

We put the proposition to the patient and explained that this was experimental and might not work and if that being the case I would proceed to a conventional open operation. He agreed.

So this was what we did. Michael did the track, dilated it and passed a 1.0-cm tube into the kidney with very little bleeding. Twenty-four hours later the patient was taken back to X-ray, I removed the tube and passed an ordinary cystoscope down the naked track and into the kidney collecting system. To my relief, I could see the stone quite clearly. It was a yellow crystalline aggregation of calcium oxalate sparkling in the intense illumination of the endoscope light and looking like a spoonful of granulated brown sugar on a bed of porridge. I then passed a small wire basket down the cystoscope into the kidney, caught the stone and extracted it down the track. As the stone emerged it was the first time in my life that staff in the X-ray room broke into applause! The tube was replaced and as there was negligible bleeding it was removed the following morning and the patient went home the same day.

We were delighted and so was the patient and thereafter our professional lives changed completely. This was truly a Sea Change in our efforts to minimise surgical damage to a patients normal tissues and effect the required therapeutic result.

This epitomised what I had been trying to achieve over two decades of surgical practise the minimisation of surgical trauma. From now on, all our efforts were devoted to developing instrumentation and techniques to deal in a similar way with all manner and types of stone and other renal conditions. We performed a number of similar operations and presented our results at the BAUS (British Association of Urological Surgeons) meeting in Liverpool in 1980. Some colleagues were encouraging and impressed. Others were a little deprecatory and regarded the whole thing as a stunt of limited applicability and NOT renal surgery.

It was following this that I contacted several of the surgical instrument manufacturers who over a number of years had become personal friends. I wrote to companies such as Messrs Olympus from Japan and Essex, Storz and Wolf from Germany; also to Messrs Thackeray in the UK to see if they could produce instrumentation more suitable for these procedures than a cystoscope [Fig. 19.2].

What we were mostly lacking was purpose built endoscopic instruments of lesser calibre but functionally adequate dimensions

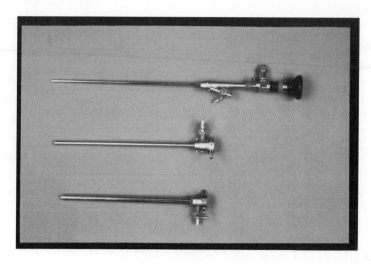

Fig. 19.2. Standard cystoscoper.

so that we could manoeuvre them atraumatically around inside the kidney and gain vision and manipulatory access to all areas of the intrarenal collecting system, the pelvis and calyces of the kidney — some being quite difficult to get to.

Secondly, we were restricted by the size of stone that we could deal with because we could not remove anything larger than 1.0 cm down the 1.0 cm track which we could not safely enlarge. Thirdly, we needed some mechanism by which we could fragment large stones into a size that were possible to remove.

In the next two years, the manufacturers were amazing [Fig. 19.3]. They firstly produced endoscopes with both solid rod and flexible optical systems that could look around the bends and nooks and crannies in the collecting systems. Secondly, they produced disintegratory instrumentation which allowed stone fragmentation to suitably sized smaller particles using ultrasonic probes and shockwave electrical discharge probes both of which had the desired effect. We were then after considerable experience able to deal with practically any stone that came our way. We simply shot ahead and by 1983 we had treated almost 300 patients. We had some interesting publicity. The BBC invited me to do several

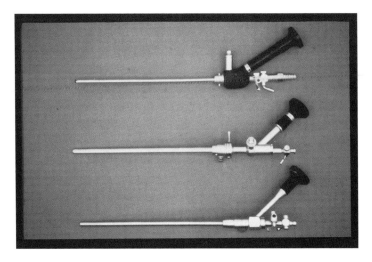

Fig. 19.3. Three types of nephroscope.

programmes with the Producer Fiona Holmes in the "Your Life in Their Hands" series specifically on the treatment of renal stone disease ranging from open surgery with hypothermic preservation of function through to percutaneous endoscopic stone removal. These programmes were apparently successful and brought useful attention to the Institute of Urology and St Peter's Hospitals. Fiona Holmes asked me what we called the endoscopic method we had devised. I said 'Minimally Invasive Surgery.' She said 'You can't call it that, people won't know what you are talking about. I think it should be called "keyhole surgery."' Both names stuck.

By then, word had spread around and other departments in Europe and the USA who were off the mark. In 1982, I thought it would be a good idea to host a meeting under the auspices of the Institute of Urology in London to meet up and discuss our various techniques. I wrote around to colleagues in Germany, France, Sweden, Austria, Italy and the USA etc. suggesting we could meet in London in 1983, expecting a small response. To our surprise and ultimately alarm we had nearly 300 acceptances. We were then under considerable pressure as week by week a further 20–30 attendees signified their intention of coming. This was way beyond

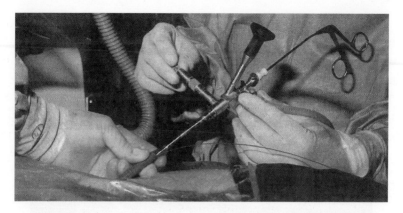

Fig. 19.4.   Endoscope, nephrolithotomy, St Paul's Hospital, 1980.

our capacity to pack everyone in at the Institute of Urology and we had to move the venue to the Institute of Directors then at Centrepoint in Oxford Street.

At the meeting, we were smugly satisfied to find that we had at that time the largest number of endoscopic renal stone treatments in the world [Fig. 19.4]. Others hastily caught up, especially the Americans, all eager to claim precedence. As usual, one is never unique and others had been thinking along similar lines. One of the delegates was a radiologist from Stockholm, Professor Fernstrom, who a year or so before had removed some small kidney stones under radiological control but had not used an endoscope to visualise the stones but extracted them down a narrow track using a basket passed into the collecting system. He was warmly welcomed to the meeting — it is interesting how similar techniques occur in different countries at the same time! Secondly, Professor Peter Alken from Germany had removed residual calculi as a salvage procedure from several kidneys that had had open operations and been left with an ordinary drainage tube nephrostomy and down which he had passed an endoscope to remove stone fragments that had been left behind.

Thus, it seemed to me that our technique was truly the first to make a primary definitive, dilated and elective track into a kidney and use an endoscope intrarenally to remove stones from a previously unopened collecting system.

At the end of the meeting which we had intended as a one off situation, colleagues from the various continents decided that this association of likeminded surgeons should be perpetuated in the nature of a Scientific Society and that we should hold annual meetings at different venues around the world. It was decided to name the society the 'Endourological Society' and I became the first Chairman with a remit to get the society active and move it along.

The Society next met the following year in Vienna organised by Professor Michael Marberger and so on annually in many different venues and is still very active. It is worth recording that all our clinical work on endoscopic stone removal took place in the X-ray Department at St Paul's Hospital. Initially, I was keen to extend this work to the Department at Barts and this would obviously require liaison with the Department of Radiology. There was one radiologist concerned with urological problems at the hospital to whom the project was presented. This person was not prepared to provide the necessary instrumental tracking facility that we had at St Paul's. I discussed the problem with the Chief of Radiology at that time and it became obvious that such assistance would not be forthcoming so no formal endoscopic urology service for renal stones took place at this hospital until a little later when another Consultant Urological colleague, Hugh Whitfield, taught himself how to do the necessary tracking procedure without a Radiologist.

This lack of enthusiasm to innovate sometime appeared endemic at this hospital. Apart from a few very active departments there appeared to be a degree of self-satisfied inertia around which could partially explain the subsequent demise of Barts as an individual premier General London medical and teaching institution active in all disciplines. Now Barts after several resisted threats of closure just survives as a major regional cardiac centre. All other general activities have now been subsumed to the Royal London Hospital in Whitechapel.

All this new method of working obviously took up a considerable amount of time at St Paul's (Dr John Samuel anaesthetist became expert at managing these patients [Fig. 19.5]). This was coupled with the enormous help and enthusiasm of my then chief

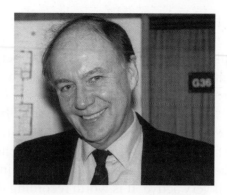

Fig. 19.5.   Dr John Samuel, Consultant Anaesthetist.

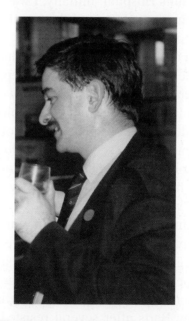

Fig. 19.6.   Ron Miller, Senior Lecturer.

assistant at the Institute, Mr Ron Miller [Fig. 19.6] who proposed that we should run a series of courses for other surgeons in this country and occasionally from Europe to teach the principals of percutaneous renal surgery. This evolved into a complex activity with images transmitted from digital cameras mounted on the

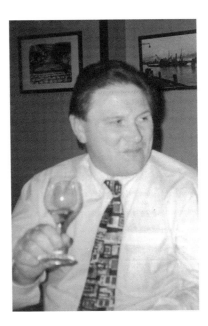

Fig. 19.7.   Stuart Greengrass, Technical Director Olympus Ltd.

endoscope being passed to VDUs in the viewing theatres but more importantly removed the need for us ever to squint with eye to endoscope optic again! Each course comprised about 30 surgeons — see copy of brochure; Appendix 1.

We also arranged with the help of manufacturers such as Mr Stewart Greengrass of Keymed to set up practical hands on workshops utilising isolated pig kidneys held in special frames. We placed simulated stones of various materials into the kidneys and the instrument companies provided complete sets of equipment for the attending surgeons to practice stone manipulations and stone extraction from these kidneys [Fig. 19.7].

To demonstrate the technique of making the access track Michael Kellett and Ron Miller helped by our Unit Technician, Larry Watkinson set up an ingenious simulation using a butcher's pig loin with the kidney intact in the perinephric fat. This when placed on a normal X-ray table and towelled up, when screened looked surprisingly like the lower chest and loin in the human situation with the kidney embedded in its fatty capsule. The collecting system was filled with contrast from the ureter and the attendees could then practice using a needle and dilators to make a suitable track under X-ray control. It worked splendidly, the only down side being the need to obtain and store 300 pig kidneys and 70 pork loins for each course. Our course registrars and helpers were sent out all over London to obtain these useful bits of offal over a number of weeks. All was well until disaster struck about 10 days before one course with failure of the refrigerator in which these articles were stored and which rotted. There was then a panic and registrars and any other available members of staff were sent out to scour the butchers of London to find replacements which was successful just in time.

I often wondered if this sudden surge in our requirements caused significant distress to the restaurants and hostesses of London. None was recorded.

These courses became well attended and continued for several years. Not only did we demonstrate nephroscopy, but also other forms of endoscopy and instructed attendees in the use of newly developed instruments such as flexible and solid rod ureteroscopes for dealing with ureteric calculi [Figs. 19.8 and 19.9]. For more details, see Appendix 1. At the same time that we began with these courses, I was still attending the meetings of the other little society that we had started, namely "The Intra Renal Society". I had also

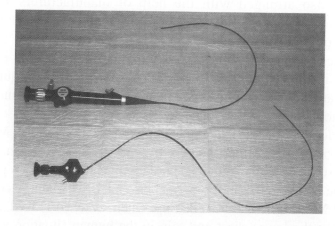

Fig. 19.8.   Flexible ureteroscopes.

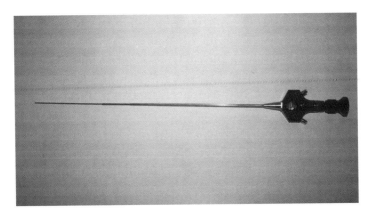

Fig. 19.9. Solid rod 3.0 mm diameter ureteroscope.

edited a book on the various open surgical procedures being carried out by our members in Europe which was published in 1984.

A very interesting topic which had been mentioned at our Society meetings over the previous 2–3 years had been the experimental application of extracorporeal shockwaves in attempts to shatter renal calculi *in situ* in involved kidneys.

While we sat back and self-congratulated on our percutaneous efforts, we were soon to be smartly overshadowed!

Chapter 20

A Slight Deviation — Gall Stones

At St Paul's Hospital, we had a close liaison with the nearby Middlesex Teaching Hospital and one day a discussion took place between Radiologist Mike Kellett and Dr Bill Lees a Radiologist at the Middlesex concerning a patient who had recently presented there. She was an unfit ill old lady in her 80s suffering from an inflamed gall bladder full of pus which was caused by a gall stone obstructing her bile duct. Dr Lees under ultrasound guidance had managed to needle the gall bladder under a local anaesthetic and drain the pus filled system. He was then faced with the problem of dealing with the obstructing stone as the patient was unfit for a general anaesthetic and the stone was too large to be removed from further down the bile duct by retrograde flexible cholecystolithotomy and basketry.

In consultation with Dr Kellett, it was suggested that with our experience of dealing with renal stones we might be able to help endoscopically. Mike asked me to assist and under local sedation I was able to pass a ureteroscope down the drainage track, into the gall bladder and on down the very dilated bile duct, see the stone and remove it. All settled quickly and the patient was discharged home after a few days.

Through this success and our enthusiasm for another application of a 'Minimally Invasive' technique, I became friendly with colleagues in the Department of Gastroenterology at the Middlesex headed by Dr Peter Cotton together with the Hepatobiliary Surgeon, Christopher Russell. With this team, we discussed the possibility of treating stones in the gall bladder endoscopically. Work commenced using two animal models and Mike Kellett and Dr Lees worked out a system for radiologically passing a needle and guide wire to develop a track which then allowed the surgeons to pass either a nephroscope or ureteroscope into the gall bladder and access the bile duct. This worked quite well and we turned our attention to patients suffering from gall stones either removing them intact or breaking them into smaller pieces for removal. We also passed endoscopes down the bile duct to retrieve any obstructing calculi. This became quite a successful procedure and we all combined to set up a number of demonstration meetings which were presented to audiences on TV screening. Christopher Russell and I operated on over 100 patients with quite good results [Fig. 20.1]. One meeting was so large that we transmitted demonstrations to an audience at The Royal College of Physicians from patients in the Middlesex Hospital and the London Clinic. Unfortunately, there were two problems with this approach.

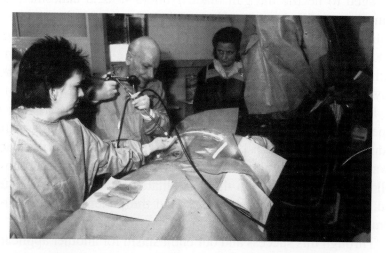

Fig. 20.1.   Operating endoscopically for gall stone removal.

Firstly, gall stones tended to recur more frequently than renal stones. We biopsied the gall bladder lining and noted that patients with a small deposit of cholesterol on the wall were prone to recur whilst those with a smooth lining remained free from recurrence. Secondly, temporary leakage of bile from the puncture in the gall bladder took longer to close and patients were sent home with small drainage tubes to be removed later on when the leak had sealed.

We also thought of applying the lithotripter (see later) to fragment the stones but this was not successful which because of their waxy nature they would not shatter unlike renal stones.

Finally, these attempts were brought to a halt when in 1986 Professor Mouret from Lyon, Professor Dubois from Paris and Professor Perrisat from Bordeauxl in France at the same time demonstrated that it had now become possible to excise the whole gall bladder containing stones transperitoneally with a laparoscope thus solving the problems of recurrence and biliary leakage. We had initially felt that it was important to retain the gall bladder as there was some evidence that patients more frequently developed colonic cancer after cholecystectomy due to the constant trickle of neat bile into the gut although this has not been confirmed.

This latter technique has now become the routine method of treatment with patients being far less traumatised than by the previous open operation and requiring only a 48-hour stay in hospital instead of 7–10 days. So, surgical science took another spectacular leap forward demonstrating again the thinking that was occurring at that time to many surgeons and radiologists in different specialities. So, back to Urology. Incidentally, it was suggested by one of my colleagues on the Council of the British Association of Urological Surgeons that I should be struck off from this organisation for ignoring a rule that a member should perform nothing but Urological surgery. I was not aware of such a ruling which appeared to effectively prevent any lateral thinking between specialities. Nothing became of this caveat!

Chapter 21

The Dornier Extracorporeal Lithotripter, The Academic Unit, University of London and Retirement from Barts

Back to Urology!

Two of the founder members of the Intra Renal Society were Professor Pitz Eisenberger and Professor C. Chaussy who were working at that time in Munich, Germany in the Department of Professor Schmidt.

At our society meeting, they had presented some of the preliminary work on the experimental destruction of renal calculi and other materials by a non-contact method of using externally developed shockwaves transmitted through a water medium to access the stone.

The concept had started with a conversation between Eisenberger and a member of the Dornier Aircraft Company in Germany who had mentioned that externally induced shockwaves experienced when high speed aircraft encountered particularly dense rain clouds, set up shockwaves at the aircraft's surface that were then transmitted to the interior and caused significant damage to electrical equipment. Eisenberger asked if it was considered that shockwaves had enough power to fragment materials such as renal calculi. The engineer said 'I don't know, why don't you try the experiment' which Eisenberger and Chaussy did in Professor Schmidt's Department in Munich, and finding it could be successful on the bench, developed an experimental shockwave apparatus to fragment implanted stones in the kidneys of anaesthetised dogs.

Eisenberger and Chaussey presented their results to our small club and had just published their preliminary papers in this subject.

The buzz in the meeting was that these men were slightly off their heads but who in the event had the last laugh and whose technique was used in patients in 1981 and succeeded brilliantly. We all changed our minds very rapidly! We could immediately see that this was set to change the whole face of renal stone treatment, which of course it has.

One of the repercussions of all this was the fact that this was going to be of outstanding significance to the organisation of renal stone treatment in the UK and worldwide. As St Peter's Hospital had originally been designated at its foundation as 'The Hospital for the Treatment of the Stone,' I felt it was important to invest in a lithotripter as soon as possible.

The Dornier company commenced manufacturing these machines for clinical use in 1981 and they became available for purchase.

When I visited this machine in Munich, it was obviously good and was going to have profound significance for the whole treatment of renal calculus disease. One could not get much more minimally invasive than with a technique which required no wound incision at all! I talked to the administration at St Paul's and they agreed that I should make an approach to the Department of Health for assistance in purchasing a unit which then cost about 1 million pounds.

I went to the appropriate department at the Elephant and Castle headquarters of the NHS and was received by three administrators and explained the situation. Within an hour, there was a flat rejection of the project. Time went by and a year later, I went through the same procedure only to be told by the jovial doctor who was Chairman of the Committee that such a purchase was impossible as it was too experimental; i.e. the bureaucrat as usual knowing better than people on the ground! This was despite the fact that by this time Germany had seven of their units working and within three years had achieved treatment of almost all patients on their waiting lists for renal stone removal in the whole country! Similarly, much stone clearance was being achieved particularly the USA where in the end about 60 lithotripters were in use. Likewise, the machine had been rapidly approved in many other countries which were then using these machines. So, this quite revolutionary apparatus was not going to be made available in the UK!

Feeling more than a little annoyed that having pioneered endoscopic renal stone treatment we were in distinct danger of falling well behind many other countries. I was one day in conversation with administrators in the private sector from the Kuwait Health Office (KHO) in London and for whom I had treated a number of their stone patients over the years. I told them about the lithotripter. 'If it is as good as you say we can send an evaluation team to Munich to see what it is like.' A team was sent and instantaneously came back to say 'We would certainly purchase a unit to treat our quite numerous stone patients. We would install it in London and would you organise the running of a proper stone unit?' It was a great opportunity to catch up and we managed to come to a suitable arrangement in that I would run such a set up if they would promise to treat a certain number of NHS patients plus allowing the registrars from St Peter's to rotate for short periods through the unit to gain experience in the methodology. The KHO agreed and immediately bought a previously rundown clinic in Welbeck Street, London and within about five months in 1984 had refurbished it and installed a Dornier Lithotripter.

The impossibility of taking on another large commitment without re-ordering my life considerably was now necessary. It had recently been suggested that I might take over a vacancy as Head of the Academic Unit at the Institute of Urology of London University with a newly established Chair of Professor. I was very happy to take this on but there were several snags. Firstly, it was nearly a full time appointment with a very limited opportunity for private practice on which I now relied for a considerable part of my income. Secondly, I would have to give up the Department of Urology at Barts and now added to all this was the proposed lithotripter unit which complexed everything.

After much consideration, I decided that I could no longer do justice to Barts and I asked for a year's leave of absence to get these various problems sorted out. I also accepted the appointment to the Academic Unit at the Institute of Urology, University of London. Resolution of the primary question of a professorship was achieved by appointing me as Director of the Academic Unit without the Professorial title and enough breathing space to get the Lithotripter Unit under way.

Finally, I decided that despite working at Barts in some capacity or other for thirty three years and being extremely attached to my alma mater I would, in the interests of promoting progressive renal surgery, have to resign. I was very generously given one year's leave of absence to see if this was the correct decision and it is one which I have never regretted.

Chapter 22

Installation of the Dornier Lithotripter at Welbeck Street, London and the Stone Centre

The Unit was rapidly designed complete with a full radiological facility which Michael Kellett volunteered to establish. In the basement of this clinic, we could treat any type of renal stone by the most appropriate modern methods. There were an X-Ray room, an anaesthetic room, a recovery area, etc. All one could wish for. It was wonderful to at last work in a fully equipped facility unlike the often primitive situation at St Paul's.

This new clinic also had consulting rooms on the ground floor and on two upper floors there were about six to seven rooms for inpatient treatment.

Other events followed. I still had my consulting rooms at the London Clinic in which I had worked for 14 years. I was rung up one morning and asked if I could meet with the Chairman of the London Clinic who arrived in my rooms. He was obviously embarrassed but told me that as I was supporting another private facility in the Harley Street area would I kindly give up my rooms by the end of the month! I could do nothing but agree and within two weeks I had moved my own tiny organisation to Welbeck Street. One can imagine the complications that this produced.

Secondly, news of this wonder machine had reached the national press and hit the front page of The Times. I was asked for an interview and explained this latest exciting functional facility.

Then at some stage someone had interviewed the management side of the Clinic who quoted the prices for treatment! The Times reported that "Mr Wickham would treat kidney stones for X amount of money" without mentioning a word of this to me. This was followed in a few days by a most unpleasant letter from the President of the General Medical Council threatening that I should be struck off for advertising! I replied and explained the position. This resulted in another unpleasant missive saying that it could be overlooked this time but one more transgression and I would be out! So much for trying to push the boundaries of medicine in the UK! Now quite amusing in view of the amount of advertising of medical and surgical skills in various private hospitals and clinics all over the country. Do not be eager to be first to put one's head above the parapet.

During all this turmoil, normal operating lists and clinics were still being carried on at St Paul's and the teaching programme continued, now coupled with visits to view the lithotripter so we did not slack off!

The developers had done an excellent job in fitting out the lithotripter unit. All was tiled in a delicate blue colour and the entrance to the unit was by way of a passage that was lined by metallic silver coloured panels. The whole effect was totally 'Star Trek'. We set to work with enthusiasm and during the first year of running treated over 1000 patients by the different methods available.

It is worth describing the lithotripter in some detail [Figs. 22.1–22.3].

It consisted firstly of a bath a little larger than a normal domestic one in stainless steel. At the base of the bath, an electrode was situated in a parabolic reflector rather like a car headlight which produced the necessary shock waves. The bath was filled with warm water and the anaesthetised patient gently suspended in a metal cradle was carefully lowered into position and immersed with the water covering the abdominal area. The cradle was electrically

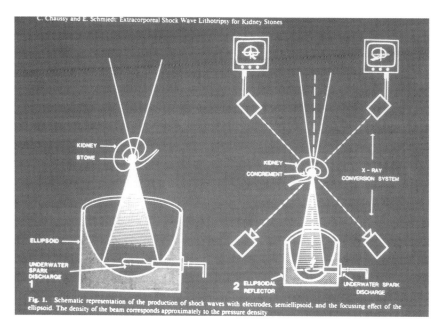

KIDNEY
STONE

ELLIPSOID

UNDERWATER
SPARK
DISCHARGE
1

KIDNEY
CONCREMENT

X – RAY
CONVERSION SYSTEM

2 ELLIPSOIDAL
REFLECTOR

UNDERWATER SPARK
DISCHARGE

Fig. 1. Schematic representation of the production of shock waves with electrodes, semiellipsoid, and the focussing effect of the ellipsoid. The density of the beam corresponds approximately to the pressure density

Fig. 22.1.   The principle of the Dornier lithotripter.

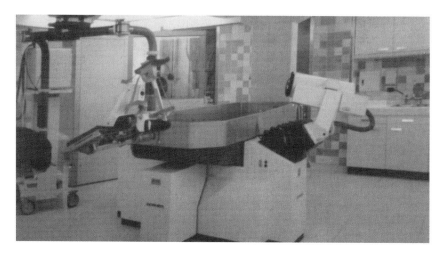

Fig. 22.2.   The Dornier lithotripter.

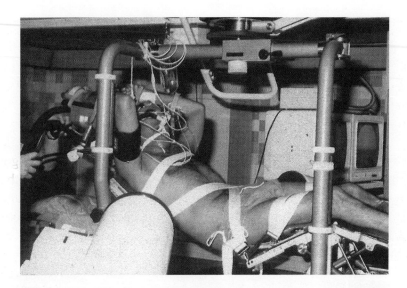

Fig. 22.3.   Patient suspended in the cradle about to be lowered into the bath.

controlled so that the patient could be moved in any direction. Once the patient was in the bath, two X-ray tubes were moved into position, one on each side of the bath. Snapshot X-rays of the relevant renal area were then displayed on a viewing screen, the stone or stones identified and the cradle moved so that aiming grids located the stone into exactly the correct focus for the shockwave to impinge on the target. When a satisfactory position had been achieved, the shock wave electrode was activated by a 15-kilovolt discharge under water and the wave focused by the reflector in which the electrode was situated. This focused shock wave then passed through the bath fluid, through the soft tissues of the patient's body to impinge on the calculus at the focal point of the shock wave. A series of shocks were then induced using on average about 50–100 discharges and the stone could be viewed to disintegrate on the X-ray screen. When complete fragmentation had been produced, the procedure was terminated and the patient passed out of the bath to recovery and then back to bed. All being well, stone fragments were voided in the urine over the next 24–48 hours and the patient discharged with minor analgesics. The anaesthetic was necessary because the passage of the shock wave was painful with a pressure of 50–1500 bar being induced. It was of vital importance that the shock was aimed purely at the calculus so that no damage was caused to nearby solid tissues such as the ribs or the lungs. Primary stone disintegration was high on average — 84%.

As we progressed, we had very few complications. Those which were most troublesome were when stone fragments became lodged in the ureter and required endoscopic intervention from below with a ureteroscope and by the passage of a temporary plastic drainage tube or stent to remove them. Very occasionally, disintegration was incomplete and we had to resort to percutaneous puncture and endoscopic visualisation to remove very large or hard stones or fragments.

Situated as we were with all the facilities we needed, we were able to immediately implement any ancillary methods of stone clearance either by lithotripter or PCN under the same anaesthetic and we only had to resort to open operation in about three or four cases in the first year of operation where stones were occasionally too hard or completely lodged in the intra renal collecting system. What a contrast to the open surgical procedures used about seven years previously!

The team at the lithotripter centre became first class — both doctors, nurses and technical staff. The medical resident staff were headed by a highly capable Australian, Senior Registrar, David Webb, in London for two years to gain urological experience and the Institute lecturers and registrars provided total backup as required. The nurses became expert at the delivery of pre- and postoperative care and the technical staff were exceptionally helpful. The whole ambiance was one of enthusiasm and excitement. We worked very long hours determined entirely by the needs of the patients and if we were required to carry out ancillary procedures we occasionally used to continue until 8.00 pm or even 9.00 pm until the job was done. I have never before or since worked in such a happy atmosphere with no complaints that I knew about with regard to the often heavy workload we experienced. It was like the old Firm system at Barts. Everyone was competent at their occupation and was enthusiastic to make it work [Fig. 22.4].

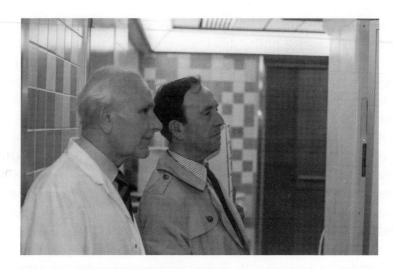

Fig. 22.4.   A more relaxed form of renal stone surgery witnessing the control panel and X-ray.

I now had my new consulting rooms on the ground floor of the Clinic and secretarial help with the documentation. The news of the success of the lithotripter spread and the NHS finally decided to finance the running of a second Dornier at St Thomas's Hospital, but even this one was purchased by BUPA a private organisation. This started working 9–12 months after we had been running.

The changes that all this produced in my personal life were considerable. Firstly, the long hours and volume of work made it impossible to travel up and down to Surrey each day and it was necessary to seek more local accommodation and I found a small flat just north of Regents Park. I got home when I could during the week and usually all the weekends. Here, I was at the age of 54 a fully trained surgeon using very few of my skills and moving over to an entirely alien process. The endoscopic portion of my work was a natural evolution of the surgical process but I was also apparently moving into an almost industrial situation with the lithotripter.

The attitude of colleagues and the profession was ambivalent. Some were intrigued by this sudden change and interested in how it was all going to end up, some were impressed by the technical success of the procedure and were encouraging.

Alternatively, an element was critical. I was thought to have become a bit of a maverick, and almost hoodwinking the patients with what seemed to be a rather sophisticated 'Black Box' piece of machinery. The fact that it was based in the private sector and worked well was an anathema to some. I had a few comments from my old colleagues at Barts implying that I was deserting the hospital when it needed support as it was at about this time being threatened with complete closure by the then current Minister of Health. I could not visualise how one could have achieved what we had now done occurring at Barts Hospital having experienced the inertia with which other innovative projects had been received.

I may also be wrong but I felt that the Department of Health was a little piqued that this monster which they had turned down had become successful and I have already mentioned the attitude of the General Medical Council.

The fact that this machine had been taken up so rapidly around the world confirmed to me that I had probably made the right decision but I had more support from colleagues and organisations abroad and the encouragement in this country was rather lukewarm. I don't know what the council of the Royal College of Surgeons thought about all this but I was awarded the James Berry Prize of the College in 1985. The citation being 'For his International contributions to renal stone surgery, his pioneer work in the field of percutaneous nephrolithotomy and his postgraduate teaching and training of urological specialists which has done much to improve the outlook for patients suffering from the stone.' Not too bad on balance, I suppose!

The hunt for an NHS lithotripter, however, continued with the more forward looking attitude at St Peter's and the Institute. In the end, after three years, we finally achieved the placement of a second generation Wolf machine at St Paul's where it was designated as the North East Thames lithotripter unit.

Personally, I was much enjoying my new appointment at the Institute of Urology. Somehow, finance was found to appoint two senior lecturers and four lecturers to form the basis of the Academic Unit. The teaching was all postgraduate and the partial aim of the unit was for the academic incumbents to be shielded from direct day to day clinical responsibility to concentrate on developing research programmes with a view to achieving, if possible, a Master's degree in Surgery a similar situation to that which I had been afforded by Professor Eiseman in Lexington, USA.

Chapter 23

Minimally Invasive Surgery and the Organisation of the Academic Unit

The 10-year period following the establishment of the Academic Unit was probably the most satisfying and professionally pleasant of my whole life.

I was able to carry on with my own Urological lists and X-ray meetings at St Paul's. At the Lithotripter Clinic, there was considerable activity and with a combination of the two units it was possible to pursue a course of clinical practice which gave me and my colleagues considerable experience in all aspects of urological stone surgery. As I have remarked, we occasionally worked until 9 o'clock at night to finish a procedure. There was no managerial interference and we just treated patients on the basis of clinical need.

At the beginning of all this activity, the Academic Unit was now situated at the Shaftesbury Hospital in Shaftesbury Avenue, London and which had been the old French Hospital built in 1874.

It was amalgamated with the St Peter's Group in 1969 to provide among other activities a basis of an attempt to provide an academic facility for postgraduate urology and nephrology in the capital.

To paint a brief picture of the Shaftesbury Hospital. It was based on a Victorian structure built at the end of the nineteenth century for the treatment of French nationals in London and was then staffed by dedicated French speaking medical personnel. It was placed on the east side of the north end of Shaftesbury Avenue. Nursing had been carried out by a staff of nuns, but of which order I can find no information.

It was a charming building, the major architectural attraction being a magnificent central staircase walled entirely from ground to the fourth floor by white and green ceramic tiles. It originally supplied outpatient facilities on the ground floor and on the first floor was an operating suite. The second and third floors were devoted to wards and the top floor to staff accommodation.

When the Institute of Urology was installed, the ground floor was converted to administrative offices, outpatient clinic and X-ray Department. The first floor was converted into more offices, conference room and a new operating theatre. The second floor was given over to adult ward facilities and upwards the floors were given over to paediatric outpatients and inpatient wards. All these facilities were open to the consultant staff of the St Peter's Group who could arrange their own lectures and demonstrations as required. These were both urological and nephrological.

At some stage in the conversion, someone with insight had purchased or leased another house fronting onto St Martin's Lane, but backing onto the hospital which was taken over and converted into the Dean's office and offices for the secretaries of the Institute, but most importantly for a modern lecture theatre seating about 50 persons with full audio–visual facilities and video connections to the operating suite so that students could view live theatre activities from the lecture theatre.

For the Academic Unit, I was allotted a pleasant office on the first floor overlooking Shaftesbury Avenue with an adjacent conference room and there were further offices for the various lecturers along the corridor with a laboratory at the end.

For the first time in my professional life in the UK, we were given reasonable facilities without having to fight for them as had been my initial welcome to the Barts department! It all became a very viable and a more or less adequate but not plush venue to work. I met two Americans early one morning as I arrived at the front door. One saying to the other 'This just *can't* be the Institute of

Urology.' — it was! The Institute was unusual as it was administratively part of London University, although its teaching facilities were embedded in the clinical activities of the St Peter's Hospital Group and the Academic Unit was supposed to develop the educational side of the hospital activities.

In all this, I was strongly supported by the administration led by Mrs Janet Wolfinden who I think regarded our antics with some amusement but was always willing to support some of the wilder ideas. I had no written remit as to what we should be doing and had to make things up as we went along. Previously, teaching had been performed by various members of the group's consultants giving lectures on their particular expertise, there being no means by which they could perform practical demonstrations apart from having a few visitors to their operating sessions. I had no particular administrative contract and as far as I could work out it was purely left to me to try design some sort of quasi clinical/academic facility for the St Peter's Group. Ultimately, I roughly worked out that my personal activities should be threefold. Lack of administrative training often led to me making stupid mistakes which could have been avoided, but I tried to distil my own activities as follows:

(1) To promote practical teaching courses for consultants who were already practising as Urologists and senior trainees who were in the process assuming Consultant appointments.
(2) To develop and improve on existing surgical procedures with the necessary facilities and instrumentation to make them more useful and viable in a normal clinical setting.
(3) To investigate and if possible develop *entirely new* instrumentation and procedures and bring them to a level satisfactory for full clinical implementation.

Whether I succeeded in these aspirations I could only guess. We proceeded from week to week in a rather ad hoc manner which I am sure would have been jumped upon by the administrators of the present managerial structures that my successors have now had to endure.

In all these endeavours, I was tremendously supported by all the lecturers and other members of the consultant staff at St Peter's.

The first function in relation to activity no. 1. The current teaching of extant procedures was conducted by various courses in different aspects of clinical urology, see Appendix 1. My own topic unsurprisingly was to develop the treatment of renal stones and was usually served by a course of two or three days' duration. On day one, a series of talks was given in the main lecture theatre by various members of staff on their specific topics. The surgeons talked about their techniques. The radiologists, led by Michael Kellett, presented the latest radiological facilities and techniques starting with X-ray diagnostics, followed by the developing processes emerging in diagnostic ultrasonic and then intraoperative and interventional radiation methodology. The pathologists would contribute material to the main subject under consideration in relation to the bacteriology and histology related to the conditions under discussion.

The nephrologists would step in and relate how surgical activities and medicine interlinked especially in relation to the efforts produced by surgery on renal function and also gave talks on chronic dialysis and transplantation.

Day two would be devoted to practical surgical demonstrations of the subjects considered on day one. We were fortunate in being able to transmit images from the operating theatre of both open surgical procedures and often more importantly give the endoscopic view of what was going on during such manoeuvres all with two way conversation. These would be full morning and afternoon sessions. After these procedures, the operating surgeon would come to the lecture theatre to discuss what had occurred and carry out a question and answer session with the audience. On day three, we would have an instrumentation session when our friends, the manufacturers, would bring their wares and set up stands in the lecture theatre to demonstrate and discuss any new instrumentation. They incidentally gave us good financial support for these courses.

We tried to make the courses entertaining and comprehensive. We arranged accommodation for the attendees at local hotels. We arranged midday meals at the Institute and at least one evening a conference dinner at a hotel or restaurant nearby so that those delegates taking part in the courses could develop a personal dialogue with the contributors both clinicians and the instrument makers.

The final attraction in each course was the introduction to the talks and practical demonstrations of an internationally well-known visiting Professor and specialist in the techniques under discussion (see Appendix 1).

The effort by all concerned with these affairs was considerable and here most of the credit must go to the lecturers and office staff at the Institute. I would particularly single out our Senior Lecturer, Ron Miller, as the most important, without whose endless enthusiasm, stamina and input they would never have succeeded. Also, enormous credit must go to Michael Kellett my radiological colleague whose input was invaluable. Supporting Ron in most of the endeavours was our versatile and innovative unit technician Larry Watkinson. The success of the audio–visual arrangements was due to Ron Bartholomew, the hospital photographer and film expert. The theatres and nursing staff of the St Peter's Group gave us unending support and enabled us to do our bit without worrying that the patients would have exemplary aftercare. Finally, the office staff of the Institute and St Peter's were totally supportive maintaining all the connections and correspondence pre and post each event long before email was invented.

The courses that we ran ranged in my own field from those in open renal stone surgery and oncology treatments to percutaneous nephrolithotomy and the instrumentation for the treatment of ureteric and bladder stones.

Although I made no direct contribution, other colleagues from The St Peter's Group conducted courses in their own speciality expertise such as the treatment of urethral strictures, carcinoma of the bladder and prostatic disease both benign and malignant. These persons made their own arrangements for their courses.

The nephrologists also delivered their own programmes and the bottom line on all these courses was the considerable input of effort by many people to arrange, participate in and make the whole thing work. The courses were financially viable and made a small profit for the Institute of Urology. Patients that were sometimes involved in a practical demonstration as part of the procedures were always totally cooperative and appreciative. We often introduced the patients into the lecture theatre and encouraged them to air their observations to the assembled company. These interventions were occasionally quite hilarious and all in all we went to bed at the end of all these events usually quite satisfied but mentally and physically a little exhausted. We had numerous letters of support and thanks from colleagues and patients who had attended or been involved.

The second function of the academic unit was to promote input and evaluate the operative processes that we were using with a view to seeing how we could modify and improve our procedures.

My own particular remit was to try and improve the current endoscopic instrumentation that we were using for stone disease. Initially, we were in serious need of a grasping instrument endoscopically to secure renal stones that could be superior to using a wire basket. With the Storz company, I helped to design and produce a mechanical "triradiate" grabber that could be introduced into an endoscopic sheath and could also provide telescopic vision of the target. Storz produced this three-pronged instrument which worked excellently for securing stones of less than 1 cm in diameter. About a year after we had been using this instrument, we became much more ambitious and needed to tackle larger stones when required with the aforementioned stone fragmentation disintegrators which had become available. Thus, this stone grabber had become obsolete within eighteen months despite it having been awarded the Cutlers Company's and Association of Surgeons Prize for the best new surgical instrument of the year! This demonstrates the very rapid changes that were taking place in the surgery of stone disease at this time.

The second area in which we were interested was the design of specific nephroscopic instruments to examine the inside of the kidney. We had our own ideas that we wanted optics that gave a wide angled view of the renal collecting system with a solid rod lens system. We found that flexible fibre scopes of that era had much inferior visual capabilities. We also wanted an operating channel down the instrument which gave us a straight run to the target. This meant producing an angled offset ocular for the eye distinctly separated from the operating channel. We worked out a design and discussed it with our colleagues at Storz, Wolf, Olympus and the English company Thackeray.

There was a rapid response and Wolf produced a nice light effective instrument and Storz produced a nice heavy instrument both after about three months. Olympus produced optically the best instrument after a year. The delay apparently being because of the need for multiple consultations in Japan and thus lost much of the market! At about the same time, Thackeray in the UK produced a cheap looking unsatisfactory instrument. Ron Miller and I thought a visit to Thackeray's might be useful taking the German products with us. We showed them all to the CEO and it needed no words to amplify what was plain to see — the English product was very poor and made one realise why the English surgical instrument companies of that time were failing. The last few remarks of the CEO are engraved on my memory 'Of course we pride ourselves on our large inventory of instruments, over 2000 in our catalogue — we can even supply a Listers Carbolic Spray off the shelf.' This says it all.

We therefore turned to the Germans and the Japanese for sensible help. It was also interesting to note that the USA at that time appeared to be in some difficulty in catching up. The American cystoscopic company instruments were no match for the versatility of those produced by the Europeans or Japanese at that time.

The next steps were the stone disintegration devices. We at first had an ultrasonic apparatus from Messrs Wolf. This was a fine probe that could be passed down the operating channel of the nephroscope upon the external end of which was attached an ultrasonic generator about the size of a small coffee cup. This was awkward to hold but disintegrated large stones very successfully. It was also hard on the hearing as the generator was held very near to the ear of the operator. Several groups noticed a distinct loss of higher tone acuity as the generator emitted a high pitched whistle and ultrasonic vibration despite the use of ear protectors. As the average procedure time using this instrument was about 30 minutes, we received a generous exposure to the ultrasonic discharge.

Finally, we were given the prototype electrical discharge disintegrator which in essence was a minute car sparking plug mounted at the tip of a probe that could likewise be passed down the operating channel of the nephroscope. When activated, the electrical discharge produced a bright flash across the end of the probe and a local shock wave which when brought to the stone surface caused it to fragment. Very successful and still in use. Care was of course very necessary to avoid placing the active end of either probe against the renal tissue where it could cause significant damage but we soon became adept at using the devices safely and treated many large stones with them.

Another problem was that small stones or stone fragments dropped down into the ureter, the conduit between kidney and bladder, which has an internal diameter of about 3.0 mm. A larger stone or fragment of greater dimension lodged in the ureter obviously had to be removed and we were in need of instruments that could be passed into the ureter from above or up from below through the bladder to deal with this situation. Very primitive instruments called ureteroscopes already existed but were far too large and too traumatic to be used with safety. Once again, our manufacturing friends came to the rescue and within 1–2 years produced tiny delicate scopes with amazing optical ability. Into an instrumental probe of about 3.0 mm in diameter and about half a metre long, they managed to insert an optic, a light source channel and an operating irrigation channel down which we were able to pass tiny disintegrating probes or small stone baskets to either secure or fragment stones and clear the ureter. These were wonderful pieces of technology and we were delighted to have been offered the vital expertise and back up that we needed. They also produced similarly minute flexible endoscopes which did not have such excellent optical facilities as the solid rod instruments but their ability to work at difficult angles enabled as to access most of the areas we were concerned with and deal with awkwardly placed calculi.

So in the space of not much more than three years we were fully equipped to deal with almost all renal stones together with any ureteric stones and either extract the latter through the kidney or from below through the bladder! Subsequently, we were joined in all this by the extracorporeal lithotripter.

These were just a few of the operative devices that were produced in a very short time and enabled us to move from very traumatic open procedures to almost entirely optical operations with minimal ancillary tissue destruction!

Likewise in the radiological area, further instrumental advances were being especially tailored to the needs of the renal access puncture. Improvements were made in the dilating probes and tubes which were used to make the operative tracks. The most used was a set of graduated plastic dilators that could be threaded sequentially over the primary guide wire passed into the kidney. Michael Kellett become so adept at needling the precise area of the kidney collecting system that his port of access was usually made with just one thrust of the primary needle — contrast was injected to make sure of the location and over the guide wire graduated dilators were passed sequentially until a suitable size of track of about 1.0 cm was reached to access the stone, The second type of dilator devised by Professor Alken in Mainz was based on an apparatus similar to a telescopic car radio aerial and was a graduated assembly of concentric metal tubes which could be collapsed one into another. When passed over the guidewire, the sequential opening of each diameter of tube allowed gentle dilation of a track.

In our initial procedures at this point, a flexible tube was passed over the guide wire and left within the kidney for 1–3 days to allow the track to "mature". As we became more experienced, we found that there was little need for the two days delay and a second anaesthetic so that we proceeded to the endoscopy immediately after the primary dilatation. This worked reasonably well in most cases, but occasionally some oozing of blood into the collecting system occurred obscuring vision. A tamponading plastic tube was then passed over the last large dilator to produce tamponade and good optical visualisation produced. With this method, the whole procedure became a one anaesthetic, one operative event. Finally, as time went on we found that if the tamponading plastic tube was removed at the end of the procedure then in most cases the bleeding had already ceased and there was no need to insert a drainage tube. The patient returned from the X-ray Department to be observed for

24 hours in hospital and if the urine passed became clear they could be discharged the following day. This of course produced tremendous savings in accommodation costs. If bleeding was a nuisance at the end of the procedure we could leave a tamponading tube in place, discharge the patient home for a day or two and then remove the tube as an outpatient and a non-anaesthetic procedure. Other radiological advances at this time were the substitution of ultrasonic imaging rather than repeated X-ray exposure for the patient. It is probably worth emphasising that these manoeuvres were all carried on in the X-ray Department with the surgical instruments being brought in from the theatre which was then freed up for other use.

So, these were the types of manoeuvres and instrumentation which we were enabled to develop.

The nature and the mode or our employment at St Paul's or The Shaftesbury Hospitals gave us much freedom to develop and refine new techniques without being harassed by bureaucratic intrusion and by such things as timing, numbers, targets bureaucracy etc. Frequently, things became so exciting that the whole team would be working late into the evening or an operation list be extended across the lunch time break into the afternoon to complete a procedure and save the patient from further anaesthesia or intervention. Never did I hear the medical, nursing or technical staff complain about these rather peculiar times; maybe, I was never told! We worked as a complete team a sort of modification of the old hospital firm system described earlier and the whole objective was aimed at the good of the patient not the target figures of an overbearing administration. How is it possible to pursue this type of activity at the time of writing is difficult to conceive? Timing of working hours, working shift work and interference from administrators with their own agendas to grind did not exist to destroy the concord that we enjoyed at this time! This was trying to improve clinical medicine 'on the go' without recourse to complex long drawn out trials of new procedures. We lived by the principal that if it obviously works for the benefit of the patient and it certainly causes no harm, just do it!

The third of our activities was to encourage the young surgeons who joined us on the academic unit to have freedom to pursue their own interests. I told applicants for these posts that as they were mature men and women of around 30–35 years that there would be no restrictions or directives on what they wished to pursue. All we could offer was time for reflection followed by the selection of the candidates' choice of subject and a degree of financial support for any experimental costs that might ensue. They could discuss what they were trying to achieve either with their contemporary colleagues, the St Peter's Consultant staff, the lecturers or myself. If possible, the work should be aimed at achieving a higher degree such as a Mastership in surgery. In this, most incumbents were successful in achieving this objective.

My only prescriptive recommendation was not to select an oncological subject for study. This was not because I had anything against oncological research, but because I felt that in one or possibly two years available to each appointee it would be unlikely to produce any significant inroads into a subject that was being pursued in any number of major institutions worldwide devoted entirely to this area of activity. I did not feel that a single surgical registrar could achieve anything of significance that was not already well catered for elsewhere. I had previously seen one or two people waste much time and money on oncological projects that could never be completed and which resulted in disappointment for the person concerned and suggested that this sort of investigation would be better avoided.

This approach seemed to work reasonably well and I think that most of the members of the academic unit appeared to enjoy their time at the Shaftesbury and the Institute.

Our week started with the Monday morning meeting at 8.00 am in the conference room. All members of the unit were expected to attend. All were then questioned individually on their previous week's work and their projections and needs for the current week which I noted in a small book. I opened the discussion and then anyone was free to ask pertinent questions of the speaker. This resulted in a quite helpful grilling by one's peers often with very useful and occasional hilarious results! Anyone who was clearly lazy and not producing anything of significance was

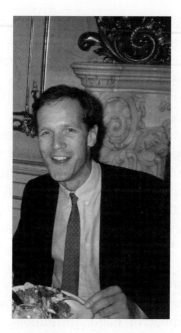

Fig. 23.1. Graham Watson.

skewered by his contemporaries. I was told in later years that the Monday morning meeting was dreaded by some — draw your own conclusions!

Arising from this arrangement a number of useful innovations emerged. One of the most significant was Graham Watson's [Fig. 23.1] on the development of The Holmium laser for the disintegration of ureteric calculi [Fig. 23.2]. One of the difficulties of using electrical shock wave disintegration in the ureter was iatrogenic damage to the ureteric wall causing a perforation which then required the insertion of a temporary stent to restrict urinary leakage. Graham investigated the properties of various lasers to disintegrate renal stones *in vitro*. He finally demonstrated that with a Holmium laser at 504 nanometres, good disintegration took place. He then performed a series of dead meat experiments to demonstrate that even if the laser was discharged directly onto the tissue, negligible effect or damage was produced. This was well worthy of clinical trial, a suitable patient was selected and the nature of the

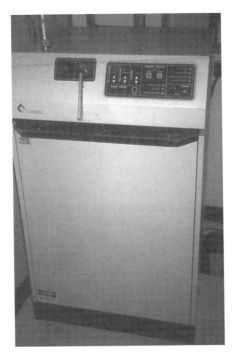

Fig. 23.2. Holmium Laser.

procedure was explained. He responded willingly and one morning in the Shaftesbury Hospital theatre we passed a ureteroscope up to the stone. A fine flexible optical fibre was inserted and a short series of laser impulses given to the stone which disintegrated completely with no obvious damage to the ureteric lining. Encouraged by this, further patients were treated and an apparatus was later developed by a laser manufacturer for clinical use.

Another avenue of treatment for ureteric calculi and endoscopic retroperitoneal nephrectomy was investigated by Ron Miller. In 1985, I was presented with a patient with a 1.5-cm stone impacted in the right upper ureter. Conventional surgery prior to endoscopic ureteroscopy entailed making a 3–4-inch incision, dissecting out the ureter, incising it and removing the stone followed by re-suturing of the entry incision. Again, it seemed to me that a disproportionate amount of tissue trauma was being caused to extract such a small calculus.

I had always tried during open renal surgery, that as far as possible the whole procedure should be carried out retroperitoneally without opening the peritoneal cavity as perforation or tearing of the peritoneum often resulted in a paralytic ileus of the gut which delayed recovery. If it was possible to work retroperitoneally down to the ureter with an endoscope it should also be possible to remove the stone with lesser side effects. For this, I needed an endoscope of reasonable calibre with a good operating channel and a laparoscope at that time looked the most useful. Passing the instrument through a small puncture in the loin I felt that I might be able with a modest amount of gas insufflation, manufacture a small pocket in the retroperitoneum in which to locate the ureter and the contained stone incise it with a long endoscopic knife and grasp the calculus. The problem was discussed with a suitable patient always with the proviso that if unsuccessful a routine operative procedure would follow.

The first operation revealed some difficulty as within the pocket developed with the gas it was difficult to identify the anatomy although I was familiar with the lay out from open surgical experience. Finally, I identified the lower pole of the kidney and traced the ureter downwards until I saw the bulge caused by the stone. All this manoeuvring was taking up some time and I did not want to expose the patient to a prolonged period of gas insufflation and anaesthesia so abandoned the laparoscope and made an incision and dealt with the stone as usual. This experience encouraged me and I had sorted out some of the difficulties by the time the next suitable patient presented. This time the procedure was much easier and went according to plan, scope in, gas in, stone out, drain in, up and about the following day.

Another case followed when I again failed to retrieve the stone due to considerable peri-renal fat. So, one out of three.

At this point, work on the more direct intraluminal aspects of renal stone treatment were beginning to take precedence and I did not attempt another extraction by this route but always felt this approach could be pursued especially with the possibility of an endoscopic nephrectomy in mind.

I suggested to Ron that it might be worthwhile pursuing this technique further either by animal experimentation or with the use of a human cadaver with permission from the local coroner's pathologist. This he proceeded to do with very good results using pig kidneys and human cadavers. He was able to retrieve kidneys retroperitoneally as a very successful experiment. It was about this time in the USA that considerable interest was being focused on the possibilities of transperitoneal renal surgery to perform an endoscopic total nephrectomy. This was achieved by Professor Ralph Clayman in St Louis who carried out the first successful operation in 1991 and we reluctantly gave up the retroperitoneal method. Mr Gau, a surgeon in India, further developed the idea of the retroperitoneal approach to both ureter and kidney using inflatable balloons to develop the retroperitoneal space rather than using gas insufflation with good success.

Another project was started by one lecturer Malcolm Coptcoat following my suggestion that it might be possible to develop a robotic type of apparatus to perform the operation of transurethral prostatic resection with greater accuracy. This project was commenced in collaboration with the Department of Robotics at Imperial College, London and will be described in detail in a subsequent chapter. Unfortunately, this project was temporarily aborted by the closure of St Peter's Hospital and the Institute of Urology but was later revived at Guy's Hospital, London. In these various ways the Academic Unit achieved a few of the goals envisaged and I believe those people who were directly involved with our activities gained benefit. More importantly, I hope quite a large number of patients were sympathetically and effectively relieved of their symptoms by our efforts.

It is now time to return to some of the more significant events that followed in my professional life.

Chapter 24

The Concept of Minimally Invasive Surgery

In 1985, I was approached by the British Council with a view to organising a symposium on the subject of endoscopic surgery across all disciplines in view of our experience in this area at the Institute of Urology. This would also entail the production of a volume of the papers presented for the *British Medical Bulletin*.

We managed to arrange the meeting for July 1986 and brought together a number of Surgeons and Clinicians from many disciplines who had recently described their experiences in this particular field. Much of the hard practical work in assembling this panel was again down to our Senior Lecturer at the Institute of Urology, Ron Miller. The many areas considered were gastro-intestinal colonic and biliary surgery, thoracic, the urinary tract, vascular, orthopaedics and gynaecology. There were also contributions from the instrument manufacturers. Other persons involved were radiologists, ultrasonographers, laser practitioners and finally members from the veterinary profession. This turned out to be a good amalgam of what was occurring in the many areas of interventional medicine at the time and was well received.

For the volume emanating from this meeting, I was asked to write an overview and introduction to the symposium for Volume 42 of the *British Medical Bulletin* which entailed doing a concise assessment of what was currently developing in these various activities and the changes that were occurring in interventional therapy and particularly in its endoscopic aspects. As I reviewed what had been presented, it became even more apparent that rather than a few independent events occurring enormous changes were beginning to overtake the whole of interventional medicine and not only surgery. Changes in the main had the primary purpose of reducing the operative pain and discomfort for many patients undergoing various therapies and inducing a much more rapid and comfortable convalescent period to follow. This tended to be at the expense of more difficult and detailed surgical intervention which was making life more complex for the surgeon but far less so for the patient.

As I began to write this present account, I got out my old copy of what I had written in 1986 for this introduction to the Bulletin and I do not think I can improve very much on it in retrospect. This is the first time that I used the written appellation 'Minimally Invasive Surgery' which I felt was a slightly clumsy way of trying to encompass this whole concept of a new approach to many areas in the interventional repertoire.

I see that there are a number of areas of speculation which have clearly not come to fruition but the main bulk of the account seems to have stood the test of time as it encompassed my thinking in 1986.

So, a number of predictions which seem correct and a few that missed the point!

The *British Medical Bulletin* is not a widely read publication and produced little reaction. I therefore submitted a précis of the article to the *British Medical Journal*. To my surprise, it was accepted and used as the first Editorial in 1987 in the Christmas edition of the Journal. Whether it was included as a Christmas fairy story I never understood but it was headed as 'The New Surgery'. Nevertheless, it caused a little more reaction than the previous piece. There was a fair amount of support but even more criticism.

As a result of this article, I was asked to give a few talks along these lines to various surgical associations where I encountered altercation with some of the members present, especially the general surgeons who appeared to resent an upstart Urologist suggesting to them what they should be doing. This despite the fact as described

British Medical Bulletin (1986) Vol. 42, No. 3, pp. 221–222

Introduction

J E A WICKHAM

Director of the Academic Unit
Institute of Urology, University of London

The attitude of surgeons to surgical access is interesting. Large incisions are applauded as bold, whilst a minimal approach is frequently denegrated as 'keyhole', timid, feeble or inadequate.

The attitude of patients is diametrically opposite. A major fear of surgery for the patient is the fear of the pain of the incision, what then transpires within the body cavities is of little interest, as long as he or she is rendered well at the end of the procedure. It has become increasingly obvious in the last few years that the patient is probably right to be fearful in his assessment of this situation and that recent events are proving that it is time for the surgeon to reappraise his attitude.

It is surely commonsense that any surgical procedure aimed at achieving a satisfactory therapeutic result for the patient should be carried out with a minimum of trauma to normal tissues and adjacent organs, although this may make the technique or operation more difficult for the surgeon to perform. True surgical skill now depends increasingly in minimising the trauma of access whilst still carrying out the definitive operative correction in miniature, often with ancillary and endoscopic instrumentation.

As a Urologist it is pleasing to observe that Urology was one of the first disciplines within surgery to attempt to reduce crude invasiveness and diminish trauma by the substitution of the notorious open lateral lithotomy for bladder stone by closed instrumental urethral lithotrity. Following the adoption of this technique the mortality for the treatment of bladder stones came rapidly down from 40% to 1%. Similarly Urology was one of the first disciplines within surgery to achieve diminution in trauma with therapeutic satisfaction by replacing the blood bath of open prostatectomy with the safer and more sophisticated procedure of transurethral resection.

More recently and in fact within the last 5 years, as the accompanying articles will show, the kidney hitherto a somewhat cryptic organ from the point of view of surgical access has come to be treated by methods which rapidly diminish the trauma afforded by open surgery with an accompanying diminution in morbidity and mortality.

In 1980 the technique of percutaneous nephrolithotomy (PCN) developed rapidly and was exploited first in Germany and the United Kingdom and subsequently in the USA. Since 1980 there has been progression from what was a significantly traumatic open procedure for the removal of renal calculi by way of a minimally invasive endoscopic method to the ultimate and totally non-invasive technique of extracorporeal shockwave lithotripsy (ESWL). The advent of ESWL should mark 1980 as one of the most significant years in the history of surgical therapy when the first patients suffering from renal lithiasis had their stones completely and successfully treated by this elegant and non-invasive method, devised in Munich in the Federal Republic of Germany.

At the time of writing in 1986 a combination of the techniques of PCN and ESWL can now enable well over 95% of cases of unselected renal calculi to be treated without resource to any open surgery and over 80 000 patients have been treated worldwide by the lithotripter and probably double that number by percutaneous nephrolithotomy. For a surgeon who has dealt intimately with the problems of urinary calculous disease over a 20 year period, the transformation of the trauma associated with the removal of a renal calculus by open surgery compared with the removal of a similar stone by lithotripsy is phenomenal. To see a 2.0 cm stone disappear from view on an X-ray screen during shockwave lithotripsy within a period of a few minutes and with the knowledge that the patient will be free to return to his normal activities within a few hours is quite staggering. The most gratifying feature of all these procedures has been the minimal physical disturbance which patients have experienced from their treatment.

It is this singular and striking lack of morbidity which has certainly stimulated my own personal thinking into ways in which similar techniques can be used, not only in Urology but also within the other surgical specialities to minimise patient trauma. I am now fully convinced that what makes patients ill during surgery is the iatrogenic damage that the surgeon inflicts upon the patient to achieve his technical aim. With renal stones the actual removal of the calculus from the kidney is but a minor part of the whole procedure. When there is no trauma of access, and the stone has been removed either by PCN or ESWL, the patient can rapidly return to his normal modus vivendi within a few hours.

To Urologists the interior of the ureter has also become accessible by means of the ureterorenoscope for the removal of stones and tumours, whilst pelvi-ureteric junction obstruction can now be dealt with endoscopically rendering the operation of open pyeloplasty obsolete. Many urethral strictures can be treated endoscopically under direct vision without need for invasive open surgery.

In this number of the British Medical Bulletin it will be seen that many other branches of surgery are rapidly adopting such non-invasive methods and the benefits of this minimally traumatic surgery are becoming evident in all specialities.

In Gastroenterology the percutaneous removal of gallstones is already being undertaken both transhepatically by flexible endoscopes and transperitoneally by solid rod nephroscopes with ancillary instrumentation. As methods of tissue disintegration become more developed endoscopic cholecystectomy is but a very short step away. An extracorporeal lithotripter is also undergoing clinical trials and it would very much seem that within the next 5 years open operative surgery for gallstones will rapidly be superseded by such techniques. Endoscopic appendicectomy has been successfully performed in Germany by Professor Semm and the Medical gastroscopists and colonoscopists are rapidly relieving the surgeons of their ulcers and polyps. It seems extraordinary that the general surgeons have not yet siezed upon the operative potential of the laparoscope. Endoscopic techniques are of particu-

INTRODUCTION *J E A Wickham*

lar value in the oesophagus again an organ previously inaccessible without major surgery. Here both benign and malignant strictures may be dilated or divided under local anaesthesia. Palliative tubes may be inserted under direct vision to restore the ability to eat solid foods, thereby providing excellent short term palliation for what is one of the most unpleasant phases of advanced malignant disease. Bleeding oesophageal varices may also be sclerosed by injection under vision without the need for the massive operation of portocaval anastomosis. By flexible gastroscopy peptic ulcers may be more accurately diagnosed than by barium studies and can then be biopsied directly. Bleeding ulcers can be coagulated and the patient treated conservatively with hydrogen ion blockers and the previously mutilating surgery of gastrectomy avoided.

An endoscopic bowel resection is theoretically feasible and we are simply awaiting the instrumentation technology to be developed for this to be achieved. It is also interesting that within the field of general surgery indirect hernial repair can also be carried out laparoscopically through a small abdominal puncture. The neck of the sac at the internal ring can be identified, the 'sac' inverted, ligated and resected again negating the need for an external and sometimes painful incision.

For the Vascular surgeon, endoscopic endarterectomy is now well in development with both flexible and solid rod endoscopes. With suitable balloon occlusion of the specific arterial segment it is possible to visualise the whole length of the arterial lumen. Coupled with the development of the 300 micron laser fibre it is now possible to vaporise arterial plaque under direct vision in quite small arteries with an access puncture of only 0.5 cm and re-establish vascular flow. Coronary artery obstruction has yet to be treated by such a technique but it will probably not be long before the vast and invasive procedure of open coronary bypass surgery will become a matter of historical curiosity, having been super-seded by balloon angioplasty or laser plaque ablation.

The Orthopaedic surgeons have already vastly reduced the trauma and morbidity of intra-articular operations with arthros-copy of the knee. Other joints have also become accessible to endoscopic treatment, namely the shoulder, elbow, ankle, wrist and hand joints.

The Chest surgeons have used bronchoscopy as a diagnostic tool for many years and are now moving on into photodynamic therapy by laser for bronchial tumours as a curative treatment. The Neodynium Yag laser is already being used palliatively down the bronchoscope to cut a way through obstructive tumour lesions and clear the bronchi to secure a palliative airway. This is obviously a technique which was not amenable to open surgery but is now beginning to give considerable relief to a number of patients suffering from terminal neoplasia in the chest.

In Neurosurgery endoscopic examination of the ventricular cavities and computer guided laser ablation of cerebral tumours through small craniotomies is already being carried out. It also seems not impossible that some sort of microendoscopic approach to the treatment of prolapsed intravertebral disc will become available in the next few years.

ENT surgeons have mastered the surgery of the middle ear and even the inner ear with the operating microscope, thereby avoiding the mutilating transmastoid approach to these structures. Likewise the larynx has become available to detailed endoscopic exam-ination and microlaryngeal surgery can now be carried out under magnification. The nose and paranasal sinuses are accessible to direct examination and limited operative manoeuvres within the sinuses can now be carried out.

Gynaecologists were early to adopt endoscopic techniques for their use and in particular the laparoscope. Professor Semm of Kiel, West Germany, has been in the forefront of the development of this technology and his paper in this Bulletin admirably demonstrates the range of the operative technology that can be achieved by this modality of endoscopy. Colposcopy again with laser assistance is changing the management of early cervical cancer.

Thus in the last 10–15 years specialists in all disciplines have begun to see the tremendous benefits to be conveyed to patients by use of endoscopy coupled with micro manipulatory techniques. That such methodology is not limited to the human species is well exemplified in the papers in this Bulletin which demonstrate the use of the endoscope in large and small animals. The therapeutic potential of such approaches within the whole spectrum of veti-nary medicine and surgery must be vast.

It seems to me that over the next 20 years we are going to see an increasing therapeutic use of other physical modalities, such as ultrasound and the laser. It would appear that the largest area of development is going to be concerned with methods of tissue ablation. It will be increasingly important to be able to break up and remove such lesions as localised tumour and to be able to coagulate bleeding vessels, disintegrate tissue and suction remove even whole organs such as the gallbladder. The chapter by Mr Bown covers the applications of lasers in this respect. All the ablative techniques depend upon the ability to administer a large amount of disintegratory energy very precisely and in a controlled manner to a point target area. Having destroyed and ablated the tissue some method of aspiration of the resultant debris will be required. The ultrasonic Cavitron appears to be the first step in this direction and is already being very extensively used for the ablation of solid tumours but only at open surgery. It would seem likely that in the next 5 years we shall see similar instrumentation developed for endoscopic use.

I think in retrospect that the decade 1980–1990 may come to be regarded as the era of the development of the concept of minimal invasive surgery. The bloody era of the surgery of Sir Lancelot Spratt and 'the good big incision you can get your head into' is rapidly and thankfully drawing to a close. It is becoming increas-ingly obvious that what makes patients ill after conventional surgery is the mutilating damage to muscular tissues, nerves and blood vessels. Exsanguination from careless surgery, literally drains away a complex body organ, the blood,leading to sequential biochemical and haematological disorganisation. Minimally inva-sive and microendoscopic surgery circumvents this iatrogenic damage with negligible disturbance to the patient's homeostatic mechanisms.

I would prophesy that within the next 30 years with immunolo-gists and chemotherapists taking over the care and cure of cancer, the interventional radiologists and the minimally invasive surgeons will conduct the bulk of cold abdominal surgery. The only remaining areas for open surgery would be those of trauma and reconstruction. It may well be that in the light of these changes our conventional training methods for surgery require a radical and rapid reappraisal, for the next generation of surgeons will not be butchers/carpenters but will be micro-endoscopists and bioengi-neers. I think it will behove the surgical profession to look well on these radically new concepts and prepare themselves for an almost total change in professional direction which will occur within a very short time span. If we do not demand such changes for ourselves our patients certainly will.

above I had had quite an extensive general surgical training before focusing on Urology.

As time went on, I began to meet more and more practitioners from various surgical disciplines who provided detailed input into what they were doing. More interestingly, it was the Radiologists who were increasingly developing an interventional interest in other surgical areas. Much success in all these endeavours depended upon the back up offered by the instrument manufacturers.

At this time we decided at the Shaftesbury Hospital that we would do our best to set up a new unit — the Minimal Invasive Therapy Unit in 1986 to pursue these methods within Urology [Fig. 24.1].

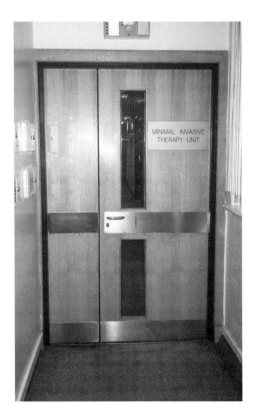

Fig. 24.1. Entrance to minimally invasive therapy unit.

Chapter 25

The Society of Minimally Invasive Surgery, Then Therapy! SMIT

In 1988, I thought it would be an interesting exercise to get a number of these people together to hear what we could learn from an exchange of views. I wrote round to a number of surgeons, radiologists and instrument manufacturers worldwide to ask if they might be interested in such a meeting. I had a good response and we suggested a modest gathering on neutral territory at the Royal Institution in Albermarle Street in London as a convenient and appropriate ground to get together. It did not seem advisable to hold a meeting at a purely surgical or radiological venue. This thought coupled with a reasonable quoted price seemed to suit but unfortunately the lecture theatre on offer could only hold 100 seats so we had to turn away quite a few interested enquiries.

The meeting was finally arranged, with much help from the Senior Lecturer at the Institute of Urology, John Fitzpatrick who subsequently became Professor of Surgery in Dublin, but now sadly deceased, and took place on 11–12 December 1989 at the Royal Institution. We tried to arrange delegate numbers into the three roughly equal areas mentioned above surgeons, radiologists and manufacturers. We called the meeting 'The Society of Minimally Invasive Surgery' with an appropriate Logo [Fig. 25.1]. We also tried to arrange presentations from all

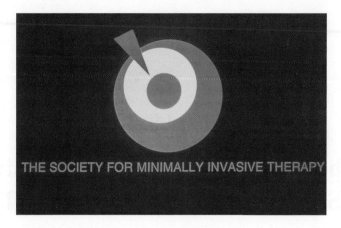

Fig. 25.1.   Logo for society of minimally invasive surgery.

the major surgical specialities and these were truly international. It was a great shame that we did not have more capacity for other delegates but we were on a restricted budget. I reproduce a copy of the programme at the time (see Appendix 2).

A number of important items devolved from this first meeting of SMIT which revealed a rapidly increasing use of endoscopic and radiological procedures and the relegation of many open operations across all specialities — far too many to itemise.

Subsequently, the effects of the adoption of these new procedures were to have a considerable impact and variation in the practice of interventional medicine in future decades and I mention a few that emerged from this meeting.

Firstly was the rapidity in recovery of the patients indicating a need for a more dynamic mode of activity in the hospital systems of that time as patient throughput was dramatically increasing and time in hospital plummeting.

Secondly, the change from general to local anaesthesia so that occasionally only simple sedation was required to permit a procedure.

Thirdly was the change from inpatient to outpatient procedures and the decreasing requirement for hospital hotel facilities.

Fourthly was the increasing importance of the Radiologist to many surgical processes and not just in diagnosis but as an interventionist.

Fifthly, there was a very obvious need for the establishment of specific training programmes in these techniques. It was pointed out that some practitioners were enthusiastically undertaking procedures with which they were already familiar as an open operative procedure but were quite out of their depth with the use and the range of instrumentation that had become rapidly available — often with disastrous results. For example, the later stampede into laparoscopic cholecystectomy.

Sixthly, it became obvious that the manufacturers were entirely willing to help in the development of new instrumentation as it was producing a boom in their sales figures plus the fact that they were gaining important R and D information at little cost direct from the Clinicians as was pointed out by one of the Speakers.

Finally, it became evident that in these procedures there was urgent need for collaboration between the various disciplines. The surgeon as the 'Omniscient Captain on the Bridge' and in sole command of a procedure was likely to become incapable of pushing all the buttons and pulling all the levers at the right time as a solo enterprise. The need for team collaboration was very much indicated and the certain fact emerged that in this new type of intervention as in a large ship one would not be able to succeed as a sole driver but would require a navigator, a signal officer and a few engineers or you would finish up with a "Concordia" type of disaster!

I found the whole gathering a great intellectual boost. One of the most important aspects that I personally experienced was the privilege of meeting and getting to know clinicians and manufacturers from all over the world at a very personal level. For instance I became very friendly with large number of Clinicians from Europe and the United States [Fig. 25.2].

I had been pursuing our speciality of Urology for nearly 20 years resulting in a degree of isolation from the main stream of surgical practice and I was once again meeting up with many very stimulating colleagues who were likewise ploughing their own particular furrows to the exclusion of the efforts going on in different areas.

To discuss at a very personal level with Neurosurgeons, Colonic surgeons, Ophthalmic surgeons, ENT surgeons etc. and exchange

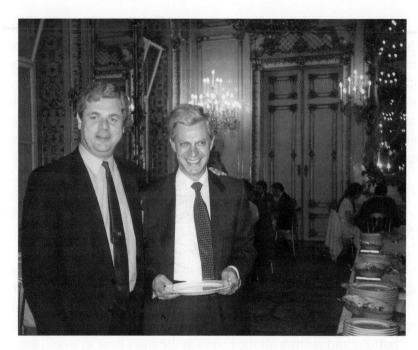

Fig. 25.2.   John Fitzpatrick, Senior Lecturer, and Professor Michael Marburger, Vienna.

our experiences was most enlightening and I saw very quickly that Urology was quite a small speciality in this whole galaxy of different activities. At the end of the meeting which had been designed as a 'one off' event, it emerged that it was the wish of the attendees that further gatherings should take place.

There was, however, a surprise in the attitude of the attending Radiologists. We had started the conference by calling it a Society of Minimally Invasive Surgeons and as the terminal discussions took place the radiologists rapidly pointed out that if such a society was to further its initial intent then radiologists would not attend a meeting apparently dedicated to Surgery. We sought for a rapid solution to this and the best that the open company could suggest was that the gathering should be called 'The Society for Minimally Invasive Therapy'. I personally felt that this sounded rather like a Collection of Homeopathists but this appellation was agreed and the society became SMIT and not SMIS and so it has remained and

Summer 1991

MINIMALLY INVASIVE THERAPY

NEWSLETTER OF THE SOCIETY FOR MINIMAL INVASIVE THERAPY

Disciplines combine at birth of society

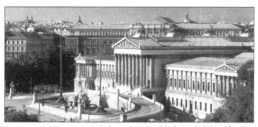

Vienna provided the venue for the 2nd annual meeting of the Society for Minimal Invasive Therapy. The meeting was held from 14-15 December 1990 and was attended by over 300 physicians and surgeons from all over the world.

Many of the world's leading surgeons and physicians from diverse disciplines have joined forces to exchange knowledge of the latest techniques of minimally invasive therapy.

This cooperation has led to the creation of a new international society and is certain to accelerate the development and dissemination of a growing body of technical expertise, offering patients the benefit of therapy with minimal trauma.

The new society, called the Society for Minimal Invasive Therapy, met formally for the second time recently in Vienna for a 2-day exchange of information and experience of a wide range of surgical procedures, reported in this newsletter.

Benefits to patients

At the meeting, the society's co-founder and President, Mr John Wickham, a urological surgeon from London, UK, said that all users of the new minimally invasive techniques immediately became aware of the advantages to patients, as well as the potential for reducing hospital operative costs.

He went on to say that although the benefits of the new techniques were becoming

recognized by surgeons, their application within other disciplines was severely hampered by the traditional boundaries between hospital specialities.

"The main aim of the society is to bring together disparate groups who are basically using the same equipment and instruments, so that we can compare experience and borrow ideas from other specialities," Mr Wickham said.

This had been the aim behind the society's first meeting which was held in London in December 1989. But Mr Wickham was now able to announce the official formation of the society and details of its membership, publications and future activities.

He told the Vienna meeting that membership was now open to clinicians and scientists from all countries, and an administrative office had been opened in London to organize and manage the society's affairs. After 3 years or when the membership exceeds 1000 members, admission to the society will only be available on a selection basis.

An annual membership fee of £150 had been agreed which would include a subscription to the society's new *Journal of Minimally Invasive Therapy*, to be published by Blackwell Scientific Publications in Oxford, UK. The first issue of the journal will be published in November 1991 at the society's next annual meeting in Boston, USA (see page 8). Thereafter the journal will be published six times a year.

Further details of the society and its membership can be obtained by writing to the Society at 25 John Street, London, WC1N 2BL. Tel: 071-430 2858, Fax: 071-861 6745. The office is under the control of Ms Fay Harrison who may be contacted at any time. This office will also function as the editorial office of the new *Journal for Minimal Invasive Therapy* which is being published by Blackwell Scientific Publications, Oxford. Membership details can be obtained from Ms Harrison and articles for submission to the journal will also be happily received at the same address.

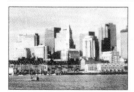

Next stop USA

The Society's next annual meeting will be held in Boston, USA from 10-12 November 1991. The meeting is being organized by the Society's President-elect, Dr Bruce McLucas, a gynaecologist from Santa Monica, California. There are places for a maximum of 700 delegates. For further information see page 8.

CONTENTS

Fig. 25.3. Newsletter SMIT society.

continued ever since, later modified by its new German administrators to 'The International Society for Medical Innovation and Technology'.

It was decided that we should have an annual meeting and as this was an international assembly (see delegate list in Appendix 2) the succeeding venues should also be international. I unwisely volunteered to organise the necessary initiatives to cope with this primary situation and get things moving and our next Venue was suggested as being Vienna. It was also decided that a simple newsletter of our activities should be written and circulated to the participants [Fig. 25.3].

I am sure it was this meeting that finally convinced me that we were in at the start of an important era in the Interventional Therapeutic experience and which was to lead on to an entirely different period of my surgical life. Despite the conventional surgical training that I had undergone and described above I was needing to retrain myself into an entirely different mode of action and way of thinking.

Chapter 26

Closure of the Stone Centre and the Move to Devonshire Place and the London Clinic

Meanwhile, day to day life had to continue as usual and in 1986 the bad news came that the Kuwait Health Office had decided to combine all its activities at the London Bridge Hospital near Guy's Hospital on the South side of the river. The lithotripter would have to move and would I carry on with the day to day running of the stone unit? This was geographically very difficult as all my other activities were based North of the River. I said this was an impossible task and I could not move around in such a difficult area once or twice a day and that I would have to give up the running of the Unit. This was a huge blow as we now had such ideal facilities well organised in Welbeck Street.

It was also suggested that I should therefore give up my consulting rooms at Welbeck Street as well as the Unit. A reaction that I was now becoming used to!

Then followed an anxious month trying to establish a new Consulting practice facility and secondly one that would somehow encompass a lithotripter. The first problem was solved by my very loyal and capable secretary, Lyndsey Frost, who scoured the Harley Street area at high speed and turned up a recently developed suite of

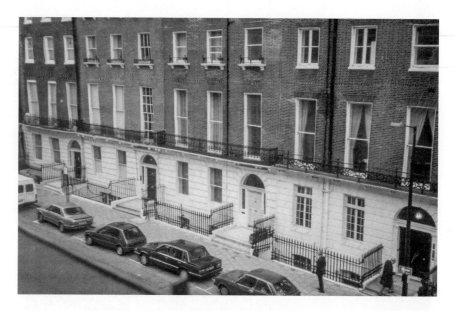

Fig. 26.1.   Consulting Rooms, Devonshire Place, London.

rooms in Devonshire Place conveniently situated between the London Clinic and King Edward VII Hospitals [Fig. 26.1].

In situations like this, you rapidly find out who your real friends are. I needed to have a lithotripter facility to maintain my stone practice and in the intervening two years since installing the Dornier about four other instrument companies had developed second generation cheaper machines. If I could access one of these where could it be installed? I went to see Mr Kent, the CEO of the London Clinic, and said 'If I can obtain one of these machines could you find space in the London Clinic to install it?' We discussed the accommodational and financial implications and he swiftly agreed to the project. Now how to finance this second machine? [See Fig. 26.2.]

I had an irreplaceable Midland Bank Manager, Eric Doughty, at this time who agreed not only to finance the lithotripter but also to help with the purchase of my new rooms. These manoeuvres were also much facilitated by an old patient of mine who had become a close friend and who was a well-recognised entrepreneur in the electronic and IT field. He suggested that I should purchase a

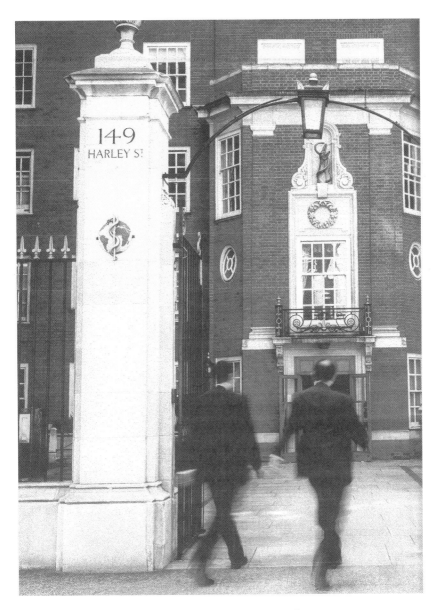

Fig. 26.2.   149 Harley Street, London.

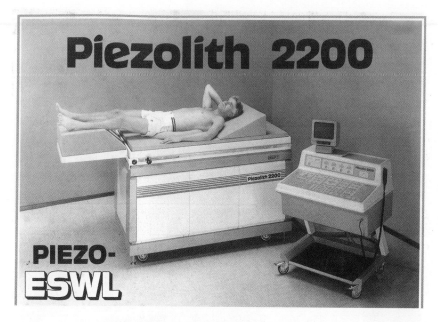

Fig. 26.3.   Wolf lithotripter, London clinic.

lithotripter with the help of some of my colleagues who generously agreed to back up the whole idea.

In early 1987, this major project was completed in just over six weeks! I had new consulting rooms, and installed a brand new lithotripter in one lightening flash. This seems hardly believable in the present day climate of risk avoidance and financial skulduggery!

Having been relieved of the stone centre commitment life started to get a little less hectic. At St Paul's and the Institute of Urology and now the London Clinic, 'normal' surgery continued with a predominant focus on renal stone disease.

The new Wolf lithotripter was an entirely different instrument to the Dornier and worked on a principal of ultrasonic induced shockwaves [Figs. 26.3 and 26.4]. These were produced by an array of small ultrasonic units arranged in a bowl shaped focussing dish about a metre in diameter and 20 cm deep at the centre of which was an ultrasound scanner. The ultrasonic shockwave array was constituted by 3000 individual tiny units mounted all over the concave surface of

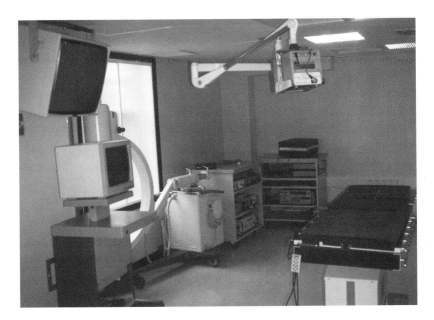

Fig. 26.4.   Endoscopy unit, London clinic.

the dish. These when all discharged together produced a focussed shock which impinged at a 2.0-mm target point. The dish was filled with warm water and the patient laid across the bowl which was built into a comfortable couch so that the appropriate target area of the patient's kidney dipped gently into the water and which provided the means of transmitting the induced focused shock wave through the water to the patient's body then through the soft tissues to impinge on the renal stone. The shock wave was focused onto the stone by means of the centrally placed scanner which identified the position of the stone on a video display unit. The dish could be moved appropriately by electrical control to access the target. The stone was then exposed to the necessary number of shocks to cause disintegration.

The major attraction of this new procedure was that it required no general anaesthetic unlike the Dornier. As the passage of each individual tiny shockwaves caused little tissue disturbance on its way to the focal point where the shockwaves summated, only a small pin prick sensation was felt. The patients suffered very little discomfort which soon settled as treatment progressed and they could follow the slow process of the stone disintegration on the screen whilst undergoing treatment!

Our first patient was fortuitously my friend who had helped us with all the arrangements for the financing of the unit and who had unfortunately developed a renal calculus quite recently and lithotripsy was recommended. He was admitted to the Clinic, the stone was disintegrated at about 2.0 pm and he then returned to his room. At about 5.00 pm, I said to the Registrar, 'Perhaps we ought to go and see Mr X.' We arrived at his room to find him fully dressed. He said 'Why am I in hospital? I have no pain or discomfort.' We could think of no reason why he was still detained apart from custom. He said 'I am sure I can go and I will take you chaps out to dinner as a thank you!'

From that day on, the treatment became an outpatient procedure and a large number of patients were so treated without complication. The percutaneous facility was also re-established at the London Clinic as a purpose built X-ray and operative suite and life returned to normal.

All this seemed very remote from my original training as a "cutting" surgeon but it was certainly the commencement of an entirely different attitude to many of the previously ingrained procedures of the past decades. The physical fatigue of long hours spent at the operating table, the iatrogenic complexities produced by some of the procedures and the time necessarily spent in attending to the patients postoperatively was markedly reduced. In other ways, the pace of activity noticeably quickened and this permitted more patients to be processed.

At last after the usual struggles, an NHS Wolf Lithotripter was installed at St Paul's Hospital as the North East Thames Lithotripter Unit and we became responsible for treating stones from this large catchment area. Running costs were assumed by the NHS and we were able to establish a Registrar level post for manning the machine coupled with a nurse and a secretary. Everything worked well and with our 'onsite' percutaneous stone facility, we could deal with a good 70–80% of all NHS referrals without resort to conventional surgery.

It was about this time that we came to witness an interesting situation developing at St Paul's. Ten years previously we had kept the surgical side of the hospital quite busy and many of the 50 available beds were frequently occupied by stone patients. Once the lithotripter and PCN developed bed occupancy fell dramatically and there were frequently a significant number of empty beds. With some nursing staff under employed, it became obvious that this situation had arisen because of these new modes of treatment. This trend brought home to me that as MIT procedures developed across many specialities this was in time to have a profound effect upon the interventional side of the whole hospital system in the UK.

Our experience with the PCN courses at the Institute had also demonstrated to me that it was going to be very important that an entirely new approach to surgical training was going to be required.

The training system that I had been brought up on and which I have described was urgently needing to be modified to encompass these new techniques. The primary training manoeuvres for coping with an intra-abdominal situation had always predicated an immediate attack by making a laparotomy incision entailing a large transgression of skin and muscle to access the pathology and perform the necessary remedial procedure. In talking about this situation I used to refer to the automobile analogy — 'To service your car and change the sparking plugs it would appear somewhat unusual to cut a large hole in the engine, cover or bonnet, damage the electrical distributor and disturb the fuel supply in order to perform a simple procedure', yet on many occasions we were still content to do this sort of iatrogenic damage to the human body and accept is as the norm. Now with the laparoscope, a degree of this consequent trauma was avoidable. Some of my professional elders regarded this as heretical especially those who had not had access to the laparoscope and its operative potential.

This also raises a very important point in the ensuing discussions that occurred with the appellation 'Minimally Invasive Surgery'. One distinguished professor mentioned that the whole matter was purely a matter of access and suggested that this affair should be called 'Minimal Access Surgery'. I strongly maintained that the access was only just the beginning of the process and the fact that access was achieved through a small entry point did not absolve the operator from further minimal invasiveness of any internal organs — a point which I defended in several rather active discussions. I would reinforce that the whole concept of MIS was if at all possible not causing collateral or any damage of an iatrogenic nature during any part of a surgical intervention. I always maintained quite vehemently that gentleness in handling any part of the human body should be the paramount intent of the interventional process. This could be so easily verified by witnessing the startling difference in recovery patterns of patients treated by the various techniques in urology of open surgery versus lithotripsy — the same thought being applied to the methods used in other surgical specialities e.g. endoscopic versus open cholecystectomy.

Having got this concept firmly in my head I tried to teach my own junior staff and numerous others along these lines. The result was that I began to be invited to give talks on all these wild ideas both in the UK and abroad. This was especially fanned by a further article which I wrote for the *British Medical Journal* in 1994 which did not always produce an enthusiastic response for example a letter that the Editor of the Journal forwarded to me (see text in Box).

While these thoughts were being expressed, the Society of Minimally Invasive Therapy was becoming established. After our first successful gathering in London, a succession of similar meetings continued to occur at yearly intervals. The next meeting in 1990 was in Vienna followed in 1991 in Boston, USA and then in Dublin 1992 and soon all round the world. Encouraged by the interest in the newsletter it was suggested that the Society should develop its own Journal and with the help of my colleagues, Malcolm Coptcoat, John Fitzpatrick, Andy Adam and our loyal Secretary, Fay Harrison plus the tremendous support of the publishers Messrs Blackwell the first edition of the Journal appeared in 1991 with the title 'Minimally Invasive Therapy' [Fig. 26.5]. As the primary Editor, I was involved in writing the initial Editorial for the New Journal and tried to encompass the thoughts that had gone into

Editor   21 January 1994
British Medical Journal
British Medical Association
Tavistock Square
London WC1H 9JR

Dear Sir

While fully acknowledging Mr Wickham's admirably pioneering place in the explosive development of telescopic surgery, I have reservations about the tone of his recent overview and futurology (Wickham J.E.A. Minimally Invasive Surgery Future Developments. BMJ 1994; 308; 193–196). His emphasis on both the speed and inevitability of predicted changes may, I feel, further excite an atmosphere of febrile urgency to embrace the new or be left behind arguably existing already and perhaps cause of harm. The reported complications of laparoscopic endeavour, some serious and uniquely introduced by the new methods, though no doubt mainly reflecting the learning curve of new techniques and developing technologies, may partly have ensued from haste not to be left on the scrap heap of surgical history. Fear of this might be fanned by over-zealous campaigning.

Furthermore, although such mishaps may be prevented in future by the thorough training Mr Wickham strongly and properly advocates, it is also not beyond possibility that much open surgery will after all to be both safer and cheaper than its laparoscopic counterpart.

In my view, therefore, a more measured assessment of what we hope to gain and what we propose abandoning (particularly in colorectal cancer resection) is desirable. After all there is almost nothing to lose, for although laparoscopic techniques achieve the desired objective with less postoperative pain and generally shorter hospitalisation, they are neither safer nor more effective in what they do. As for the economic argument, the hospital and theatres are already here and running, however inappropriate to Mr Wickham's vision of the future.

Surely in the absence, therefore, of major clinical or economic advantage, or of pressing need (and "public pressure" might be more hesitant if better informed) we should take the sound British course of quiet evolution, adopting the best as it proves itself. Meanwhile we mislead ourselves in labelling the new surgery "minimally invasive". Undoubtedly less traumatic at the point of entry, it is nonetheless only the access which is minimal, not the intervention.

Yours sincerely
Consultant Surgeon

the establishment of this new society. I reproduce some elements of it here.

> 'Our first meeting confirmed for me that it would seem that we are now entering an entirely new phase of cold interventional therapy and that the open surgery of the scalpel and the operating table are rapidly being replaced by the far less traumatic techniques of the endoscope the radio-logically placed guide wire and catheter. Over the centuries surgery has evolved in a series of quantum leaps in technology and we are now witnessing such another significant and profound change in direction.'

Historically, there appear to be a number of identifiable surgical land marks.

From BC to 1846. The 'pre-anaesthetic era' when surgery was crude and seemed limited to amputations the drainage of abscesses and removal of bladder stones.

From 1846 to 1945. The 'post-anaesthetic era' when anaesthesia permitted the development of conventional open surgery as we now know it.

From 1945 to 1975. This was the era of the advent of supportive medicine with the almost simultaneous introduction of blood trans-fusion, antibiotics and intensive care. These factors enabled surgery to expand but sometimes to undesirable levels of iatrogenic trauma. During this period it became possible to almost dismantle a patient and put him or her back together and get away with it — most times but not always! Within this period massive surgical procedures were occasionally undertaken as almost grandstand events with apparently little thought being given to the ultimate welfare or benefit of the patient. Some of the excesses of oncological surgery carried out dur-ing this period can only be deplored.

One of the practices which I always found hard to understand at this time was the practice of what I called 'lymph node chasing'! It was a sacred belief substantiated by many studies that secondary spread of many malignant tumours was by way of the lymphatics and that it was vital when the primary malignancy had been removed

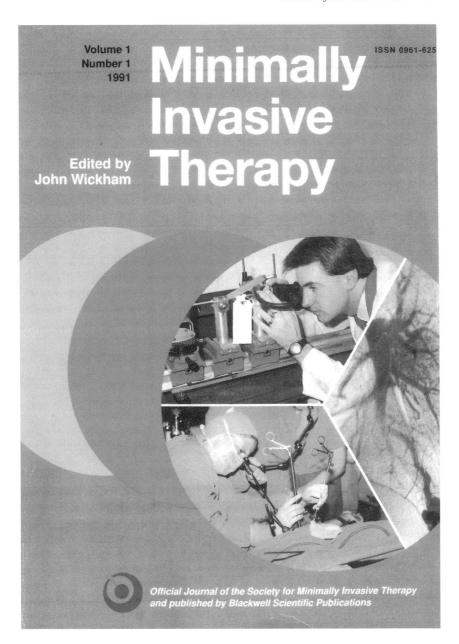

Fig. 26.5. The *SMIT Journal*, first edition.

to trace and remove any lymph nodes in the drainage area of the tumour. Some of these chases, however, reached ridiculous lengths i.e. removing all nodes around the abdominal aorta from top to bottom and even extending the hunt into the chest in the hope of removing all possible vestiges of malignant spread from pelvic tumours. Such operations became hugely traumatic events lasting many hours with patients suffering far more from these manoeuvres than from the primary tumour removal. There was rejoicing when the pathologist located a few malignant cells in one of these nodes [Fig. 26.6].

My counter argument was that as one was dealing with a microscopic disease there was little chance of locating every node involved as it was virtually impossible to make sure surgically that all trace of tumour cells could ever be removed some being outside the lymphatics and by blood spread had reached areas completely beyond any surgical access. Surely once into the lymphatic system, cells could move anywhere finally passing into the circulation and it was purely a matter of luck if one managed to extirpate the last solitary tumour containing node which could possibly contain malignant cells and which could have gone anywhere.

I maintained that you can never with any total certainty cut round cancer. You may by luck extirpate all related malignant cells with removal of the primary tumour hence the importance of early diagnosis and treatment. You may also by reducing tumour load,

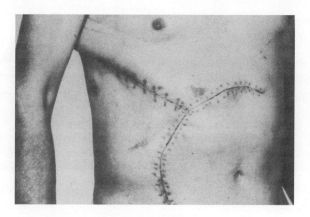

Fig. 26.6.   Incisions for lymph node chasing.

enable the patient's own immune system to cope with any strays but to delude oneself that subjecting a patient to a massive additional surgical onslaught as a means of obtaining a complete cure in these circumstances seems illogical.

I think the later treatments of breast cancer have demonstrated that a reduction in the traumatic operations of radical mastectomy which left many women with persisting disability has improved survival rates so perhaps there is a grain of truth in my argument?

Next *from 1975 to 1985*. This appeared to be the era of the development of more conservative surgery with more critical thought being given to the reduction of iatrogenic trauma.

From 1985 to date. I would identify this as the period when Minimally Invasive Surgery began to develop led by the eager cholecystectomists and the very obvious advantages of the reduction of interventional trauma began to be appreciated and brought into action.

It was also interesting to attempt to identify the nature of those iatrogenic surgical and other traumas that were bringing about so many complications for the patient? Five obvious areas can be identified.

(1) The pharmacological trauma of the anaesthetic and the analgesia required postoperatively following massive surgical procedures.

(2) The trauma of access to the target organ, quite often extensive in procedures such as cardiac, hepato-colonic or renal surgery.

(3) The haemodynamic trauma engendered by extensive surgical procedures often demanding massive blood replacement. This trauma drains away part of a vital organ which may be replaced by volume but other significant elements may still be lacking.

(4) The trauma of the definitive therapeutic procedure which compared to the ones above often appears to be quite minor, i.e. the actual removal of a renal stone from a kidney once exposed.

(5) The extensive psychological trauma inflicted on a patient both pre- and postoperatively who is scheduled for and undergoes conventional surgery.

Thus in Urology for renal stone treatment as one passes from open surgery through percutaneous nephrolithotomy to first and second generation lithotripsy, all these traumas are seen to be dramatically reduced. For example, second generation lithotripsy requires no anaesthesia, negligible analgesia and surgical access that previously required a large loin incision with significant muscle destruction, has been obviated. The haemodynamic trauma is ablated there seldom being any loss of blood during lithotripsy compared with the often previous requirement of two to three units for a difficult open renal stone operation. The trauma of the definitive procedure is negligible when compared with the multiple nephrotomies and parenchymal damage caused to the kidney by extracting stones at open surgery.

Finally, the psychological trauma is almost ablated. I am sure that there is no person reading this article who is not apprehensive at the thought of having an open surgical procedure purely because they are to be exposed to a considerable physical trauma and possibly put in danger of their life. With second generation lithotripsy this psychological trauma is removed. Within two decades, we have progressed from a situation where a patient was exposed to an extensive physical and psychological upheaval to a position where he or she is little inconvenienced, but the same therapeutic result has been achieved. Looking at other fields of surgical therapy, similar results are now being obtained.

It thus appeared that a vast sea change is taking place in the whole of the surgical and radiological environment, the mainspring of which is the appreciation of the desire to reduce therapeutic trauma by the increasing application of physical technology. It is in this regard that the instrumental engineers are assuming a vastly increasing importance in our work.

The Consequences of Minimally Invasive Therapy

It was becoming obvious in 1991 that the emergence of these minimally invasive techniques was beginning to have a profound effect in several important areas of patient management.

Hospital design:

The rapid recovery of patients treated by these techniques reduced the requirement for prolonged inpatient hospital care. Many of these procedures can be carried out on a day case or 'one night stay' basis and the need for the large 'hotel type' of hospital accommodation will rapidly be replaced by smaller local facilities with better transportation and will replace the older type of 'mega' institution.

Within these centres, the scope of operation room design will also change very rapidly from the simple concept of the operating table and scalpel to the purpose designed interventional suite containing radiological, ultrasonic and endoscopic facilities with extensive monitor displays and other ancillary instrumentation.

The type of doctor:

It would seem that the status of the surgeon as currently envisaged will be subtly eroded with increased penetration from other disciplines into the interventional process. It has been computed that there are no less than 200 allied health personnel other than doctors involved in the therapeutic process. Not all are associated with intervention, but a number of specialities are already assuming the therapeutic role previously held by the conventional surgeons. The most important of these are, of course, the interventional radiologists and it will seem very likely that new groupings will form and a team approach to therapy will emerge with the conventional surgeon comprising a smaller element of the group and which may possibly be under the control of 'a director of interventional therapy' who very probably will be a physician. In some situations, it seems inevitable that one person cannot now encompass all these disciplines. Unfortunate as it may seem, due to the complexity of new technology, the successful surgeon is almost destined to be a technologist despite the hope that he might remain the all the encompassing 'physician and philosopher who operates. The descriptive title of such an interventionist is of little consequence to the patient; as long as treatment is expeditious, atraumatic and efficient and whether this is carried out by a surgeon, a physician or an interventional radiologist is quite immaterial. It would seem that there is going to be a rapid change in the status of the surgeon as at present understood to that of one of a group of interventionists and not necessarily acting as leader of the pack.'[a]

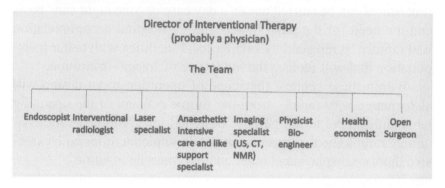

Change of speciality boundaries:

Consequent upon the above changes, the speciality boundaries will also become to be realigned. A skilled endoscopist can probably encompass the therapy of various items such as endoscopic nephrolithotomy, endoscopic cholecystectomy or endoscopic endometrial ablation. Professor Sir Roy Calne has said 'Is there any reason an expert arthroscopist needs to be trained as a physician?' It may well be that an organ specific physician will, after diagnosis, direct the patients to the most skilled 'sub-contractor interventionist' and as long as he or she is expert at his task they need not have extensive knowledge outside of their particular area of expertise.

The concept that the surgeon needs to be experienced in total operative and particularly postoperative patient care is likewise being rapidly eroded by the anaesthetists and intensive care physicians giving a further reason why the primary therapy could probably be carried out by less widely trained interventionists. These changing concepts will obviously have a profound effect on surgical training. It would now seem totally illogical to train a surgeon as a butcher or anatomical dissector but rather he or she could be

---

[a]New Players in Interventional Medicine.

primarily trained as a micro-endoscopist or bio-engineer and there should be much less emphasis on open surgery as the key discipline in interventional therapy.

The role of the health economist:

Initially, these radically changing techniques are going to alter the whole attitude of the health economist to interventional therapy. Whether health care is funded centrally or by individual insurance it would seem imperative to impress upon the suppliers of funds that these technical issues are going to require a shift of equity from the provision of long stay hospital accommodation to short stay treatment with expensive high technology equipment altering the particular nature of the interventional process. Money will be needed for the purchase and development of much more complex technological instrumentation, and less money will be required for hotel services as at presently understood. Currently, it seems difficult to persuade the financial administrators of this transference of budgeting from one area to another.

It is thus apparent that the consequences of these changes in interventional therapy are likely to be profound. Paramount is the reduction in mortality and morbidity that is being experienced by our patients and this is obviously our guiding aim. The consequential changes deriving from this seminal shift in philosophy are enormous and are only just beginning to be appreciated.

What now of the future?

As I have tried to indicate in the opening of the account of my medical training, the most important factor that was inculcated into me at all times was respect for the patient as a unique being with an individual personality. In the organisation that I suggested above, this point has been missed. I stated that as long as a patient received adequate and accurate cure for his malady he did not really care who supplied this service. This is so 'totally wrong'. Neglect of these factors of 'Continuity', 'Humanity', and 'Identity' are now being revealed as one of the major failures of the health service as we know it and experience it in the UK.

When I was a student or junior doctor, it was obvious to the patient that the paramount person in charge of his case was Dr X or Mr Y which was clearly indicated on the name plate above his bed, the clinic door and on the Physician's white coat badge. When an inpatient he or she was the doctor the patient saw on a nearly daily basis, who was a recognisable person to whom with a bit of luck you could discuss your case directly or certainly with one of the designated assistants whom you saw daily. The primary surgeon was the one who decided your mode of treatment. There was no abandonment on changing of shifts, the Sister or her deputy in charge of the wards was also a constant who would if necessary directly respond to any complaints or anxieties on a one to one basis and any nurse who demonstrated the slightest lack of compassion or care would have been sorted out instantaneously. In other words, the whole arrangement was what was known as the 'Firm System' which had evolved over a very long time. A system evolved by *experienced* physicians, and *experienced* and *devoted* professional nurses over many many years which has been dismantled by the interference of politicians, bureaucrats, and managers chasing targets and quotas but which is now being reviewed. At the time of writing in 2016, it appears that the importance of this previous 'archaic system' has at last been recognised and that the current Minister of Health and the New Director of Medical Services have suggested that such a practice should possibly be resurrected. What a surprise!

Those that are opposed to such a thesis will quote the cost implications of this older system and that the rapidly ageing proportion of the population together with the complexity of the medical process has increased exponentially and is one of a type that cannot be contained in the present economic and political climate. Both very valid points but which unfortunately miss the fundamental principal of medical care which is the appreciation of the patient as a human being with individual feelings and anxieties. Patients are not carbon copy identical objects but complex and very variable examples of biological machinery. Hard to credit sometimes when dealing with a drunk or psychopath but these latter persons are but a microcosm of the whole health spectrum.

How does one square this circle? It certainly does not improve by appointing a new Minister of Health every three to four years or a management trained hospital CEO for two years who appears more intent on personal remuneration rather than how to benefit a patient. Might it not be a good idea to occasionally consult someone who has worked or is working continuously at that sharp end of the system ranging from the GPs surgery to the outpatient clinic or operating theatre rather than a non-medical Professor of management theory who barely steps outside his office except to attend another meeting with the political masters.

Just now in 2016, there seems to be some feeble attempt at revitalising a sort of firm system within hospitals but until the burden of shift working decreed by the European Working Time directive is drastically modified I can see little hope of early improvement in the status quo and a return to Continuity which is so desired by the patient.

I fear that I am now straying well away from the story of my surgical life into areas that are not my business!

Chapter 27

Closure of St Peter's Hospital and the Institute of Urology and Transfer of the Rump to the Middlesex Hospital

The Minimally Invasive Therapy Society was up and running well. The Journal was coming out bimonthly, NHS practice was continuing satisfactorily and the Institute of Urology was still doing its best to give Postgraduate Urological education to some grades of Urologists in the UK and occasionally from abroad.

Our existence was suddenly up ended in December 1991 by the decision of the NHS to close the whole of the St Peter's Postgraduate Urological Group in Covent Garden then comprising some 200 beds and relocate it within the Middlesex Hospital in 30 beds. The contributing surgeons of the group which comprised about ten persons each doing a small number of sessions in hyper specialised areas was reduced and we finished up with five surgeons — Draw your own conclusions!

The history of the relocation of the St Peter's Group is perhaps just worth re-recording as another small facet of my surgical life. When I joined the group as a consultant in 1969, it was a busy small organisation but was performing a truly National Service dealing with complex urological problems from various parts of the country.

This facility was provided by the structural nature of the Consultant Staff which comprised Consultants from nearly all the large London Teaching hospitals each devoting about three weekly sessions to the group but in doing so provided a highly focused speciality service of their own particular expertise and dealt with complex tertiary problems referred from elsewhere.

Each consultant had his own particular niche, e.g. cancer of the bladder, carcinoma of the prostate, urethral stricture, renal stones, andrological problems etc. The theatre staff were also very experienced specialists and so were the nursing staff. At St Paul's, we worked in archaic conditions but had for years been promised re-location to a purpose built facility on an independent site.

When I joined the staff, the latest site under consideration was in South Kensington, adjacent to the Royal Marsden cancer hospital. Planning was far advanced and apart from The St Peter's Group the whole scheme was to make a large postgraduate centre with other specialities.

Despite all the architects' efforts the whole scheme was suddenly abandoned. The next idea was to place St Peter's in Holborn at the site of the old Moorfields Hospital, again planning and again abandoned. The next project was to place St Peter's alongside the London Hospital in Whitechapel. Again much planning was undertaken. Now as an added 'bolt on' to my busy schedule it was my turn to become Chairman of the Medical Committee of St Peter's. I was really 'Piggy in the Middle' of this discussion. There was enormous pressure to go to Whitechapel from two members of the St Peter's surgical staff coupled with the messianic drive of the Dean of the London Hospital who wished to build the 'Mayo Clinic of the East End'. The remainder of the St Peter's staff specifically objected because no person could afford to spend an hour and a half travelling to Whitechapel and back three or four times a week because most of their other major commitments were in the West of London. Another member of the staff had suggested a scheme whereby we went to the Brompton Hospital site in Kensington. This appealed to some members and it was left for me to inform the Board of Governors of the feelings of the staff and of the various factions among the Consultants the majority of whom would not agree to go to Whitechapel. A few things then hit the fan: I was told by the then Dean of the Institute of Urology who was a supporter of the Whitechapel scheme that I had 'poor political understanding' which was probably true but was one of the least unpleasant remarks including those of the Chairman of the Board of Governors. The ultimate result was that the Whitechapel plan was abandoned and we soldiered on in Convent Garden for a few years.

A final interesting event also occurred during my time in this office. We were asked by the Department of Health to submit a further plan of our requirements for a Postgraduate facility in Urology in London and to attend on a certain date to present them to the administration. We arrived at NHS Eastbourne Terrace on a sunny morning in May I believe, to be greeted in the waiting room by colleagues from similar Postgraduate Hospitals with the same commission. We were asked to give our presentations outlining our needs during the morning.

After lunch, we came back and we were thanked for our efforts and we were then all told that there were to be 'no further Postgraduate Hospital developments in London.' At that time, there were 13 postgraduate facilities, seven large and six small of which we were one of that latter number. 'That there will be no further redevelopment of Postgraduate Hospitals in London' was a great blow. 'The six smaller hospitals will be closed by the year 2000 and the major ones such as Moorfields, Great Ormond Street, The Maudsley etc. will be closed by 2020.'

'Postgraduate hospitals are unnecessary and expensive to run and Postgraduate medicine can be taught just as well in a District General Hospital.' So all the specialist theatre, nursing and surgical expertise was to be extinguished and considered as superfluous. Having worked in both types of facilities where one was supported by specialist junior staff, expert theatre sisters and ward nurses versus the generality of a non-specialist institution there could be no comparison. In efficiency of specific patient management and even expertise when compared to such an excellent establishment as St Bartholomew's, there was no argument.

What a waste! Another facility that had evolved and been distilled by many years of experience was extinguished NOT by medical advance or clinical judgement. We finally wound up in the Middlesex Hospital as a sort of rump. Finance and not patient's lives and wellbeing had become paramount!

So as a political and managerial decision, the St Peter's Group of Hospitals and the London University Institute of Urology was in effect closed and the dregs moved to the Middlesex Hospital between December 1991 and February 1992.

As 1992 approached so did retirement having spent two miserable years fiddling about in a very unsatisfactory environment at the Middlesex Hospital. Despite all this, the SMIT was continuing and I was carrying on in private practice.

Finally, I retired from the National Health Service in December 1992 after 37 years in the various capacities described. I was given a splendid farewell day with presentations at the Natural History Museum in Kensington when many old friends and colleagues from all parts of the World kindly took time off to attend. This was followed in the evening by a truly magnificent Dinner in The Great Hall at St Bartholomew's Hospital. I was so grateful to the many persons who made this possible.

Chapter 28

Guy's Hospital: A New Lease of Life

At the time that the St Peter's Group Hospitals and the Institute of Urology were closed or transferred to the Middlesex Hospital which completely stopped any of my further research developments, I was left frustrated with two significant problems.

One was the need of office accommodation for SMIT and the Journal administration and secondly how to manage the further development of a stalled research programme, the so-called 'Probot'.

Things looked rather glum and it was now that a colleague, Professor Andy Adam, stepped in. Andy had been one of the assistant editors of the Journal with Malcolm Coptcoat and was keen to develop minimally invasive techniques at Guy's Hospital where he was Professor of Interventional Radiology. We talked about how we could get together and work towards the development of a combined radiological and surgical MIT Unit at Guy's Hospital as I was now not employed by the NHS. I knew Professor Ian Lord McColl, Professor of Surgery at Guy's as he had been Reader in surgery at Barts when we had been appointed to the Consultant Staff in the same year of 1968. I met with Ian and presented to him the problems — no SMIT or clinical facilities to pursue our residual research projects.

Ian immediately came to the rescue. Firstly, he volunteered us an office for SMIT in his Department and in which Fay Harrison could continue with her work on the Society and Journal and also offered me an Honorary Consultant appointment on his unit to pursue any clinical research activities. He knew Andy quite well as he had also attended some of the SMIT meetings so was well aware of what we were thinking.

So in 1992 we moved the whole of the SMIT office from Blackwells to Guy's where I started working with Ian and Andy part time and unremunerated.

Another excellent event at the time was the appointment of Malcolm Coptcoat, back in London, to a Consultant post at King's College Hospital — a stone's throw away from Guy's and we could then get all together for a weekly Editorial Meeting with Fay. Things were looking up!

Incidentally, Malcolm and I performed the first endoscopic nephrectomy in the UK at Kings a month or two after Ralph Clayman had performed the first ever in St Louis, USA. So opened up another area in minimally invasive renal surgery — now routine! As I gradually settled into Guy's, Andy and I worked together to try and assemble some sort of layout and plan for a combined Radiological and Endoscopic Surgical facility. A possible site was offered and we identified and produced outline plans. Some of the other Radiologists were keen and Ian was supportive on the surgical side.

I went to Guy's on one or two mornings a week. Firstly to confer with Fay over MIT affairs and secondly to go into theatre with Ian who extended my endoscopic experience to cholecystectomy and endoscopic thoracic sympathectomy for patients with hyperhidrosis. I also had ideas for a system of hand held instruments for endoscopic surgery — more later. I was also working with KeyMed on the design of an autofocus laparoscope [Fig. 28.1] who produced a splendid prototype which worked excellently but it was then decided by Olympus that it was not a financially viable project due to its complexity so it was abandoned. I still think that if it was possible to produce extremely small digital cameras with auto focus facility then it was surely within the bounds of possibility to do the same for the operative

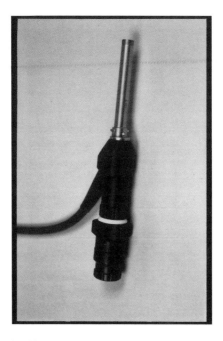

Fig. 28.1. Autofocus laparoscope, Olympus.

endoscopes now that so many are digitally based. This has I am sure been achieved.

At this time, I then turned to the possibility of resurrecting the Probot programme which went back for some time and which had been started at The Shaftesbury Hospital.

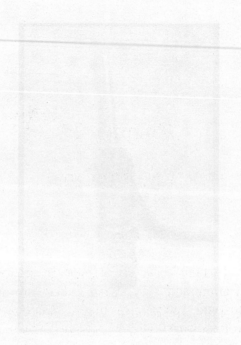

Chapter 29

The Probot

I have previously mentioned my interest in prostatic maceration which we had attempted many years previously at Barts. At the Shaftesbury Hospital, I mentioned this to Malcolm Coptcoat when the subject of robotics in surgery was being discussed. We talked the problem over and I explained to him that I had always felt that transurethral resection of the prostate was a purely mechanical procedure analogous to an industrial milling machine that removed the unwanted pieces of material from solid pieces of metal or wood. Such mechanical devices I had seen in action during my visits to the various instrument manufacturers. If this was the case then it might be feasible to build a machine that would do a similar job for more accurate prostatic resection [Figs. 29.1 and 29.2].

As I came to appreciate later, Malcolm enthusiastically seized on the idea and attacked it with his usual 'Jack Russell' tenacity. I suggested that someone with a knowledge of robotics would be a good person to advise us and I was recommended to the Department of Robotics at Imperial College in charge of Dr Brian Davies.

We went to see Brian and after extensive discussion he considered that the development of such an instrument was a possibility and immediately started off by recruiting two of his PhD students to work with Malcolm. The principal object of the whole project was to produce an instrument that would autonomously perform an operation more reliably and accurately than that which a human

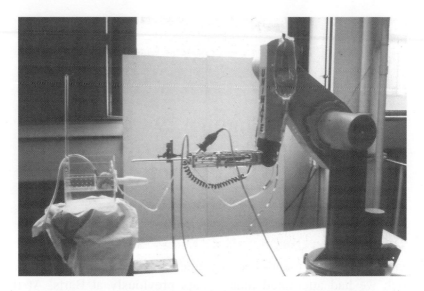

Fig. 29.1. The Probot.

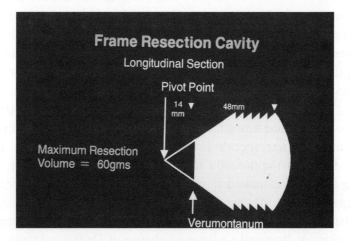

Fig. 29.2. Plan of prostrate to be resected.

hand could achieve. Time went on and the preliminary basis of the project was addressed. It was of first importance that such a mechanism should be made completely fail safe and not leave any risk at all of patient injury.

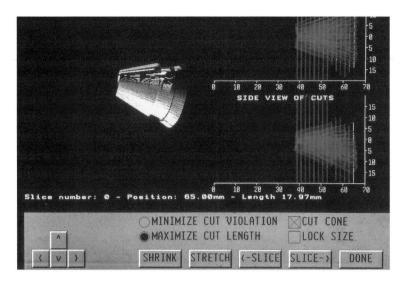

Slice number: 0 - Position: 65.00mm - Length 17.97mm

SIDE VIEW OF CUTS

○MINIMIZE CUT VIOLATION ☒CUT CONE
●MAXIMIZE CUT LENGTH ☐LOCK SIZE

SHRINK | STRETCH | ‹-SLICE | SLICE-› | DONE

Fig. 29.3. Plan of prostatic cavity to be resected, reconstructed on scanned ultrasound image.

The prototype mechanism therefore consisted primarily of a steel restriction ring which could be attached to an operating table, and upon which a conventional resectoscope could be mounted. It was decided that the principal movements of the scope would be dictated by the cutting loop of the resectoscope which would be planned to cut out a conical shaped cavity in the obstructed prostate, the base of the cone being located at the bladder neck and upper end of the prostate and the apex of the pyramid to be sited so that it impinged upon the lower border of the prostate just above the sphincter mechanism adjacent to the verumontanum which at all cost must be avoided [Fig. 29.3].

A mock-up of the whole apparatus was constructed and the movements of the scope, which was mounted at the centre of a bow shaped transverse strut that reached across the diameter of the restriction ring was fabricated. The body of the endoscope was to be attached to the centre of this strut which was then articulated at each end with the ring by a rack and pinion connection. The whole movement of the endoscope could then be rotated through 360 degrees by movement of the strut round the ring and could also move transversely across the strut by a similar rack and pinion mechanism. These movements allowed the cutting end of the scope to travel through the desired pyramidal pattern within the gland. Hard to describe!

Firstly, the endoscope was connected to a cutting diathermy electrode and moved by hand to excise the required pyramidal cavity in a series of trial potatoes. This worked quite effectively. The next step was to add electric motors to the machine to rotate the strut around the ring and across the strut as well as moving the scope in and out to produce the same effect as a resectoscope moved by hand.

Finally, the whole appliance was mounted securely on an operating table. A camera was placed on the endoscope so that movements of the resecting loop could be directly observed. All this took a considerable time to achieve — probably 18–24 months and all done at Imperial College.

It was unfortunate that at this time Malcolm had to move on to a Senior Registrar appointment at Portsmouth and the mantle of the development fell upon another talented and patient young man, Anthony Timoney, who had joined the Academic Unit at the Shaftesbury and who is now a Consultant Urologist in Bristol. When we were all fully convinced of the safety of the mechanism on the bench, it was time to assess how it would work in the clinical situation. A suitable patient came to the Shaftesbury Hospital, the project was explained to him and that we would like to try and treat his prostatic obstruction with a new robotic device. Also that we would finish the operation in a conventional manner if there were any problems. He was quite willing to participate.

The anaesthetised patient was placed on the operating table and the frame was attached. The endoscope was passed as usual and then coupled to the restrictive frame and moved by hand in the normal manner so that some of the prostate was resected all observed, under vision from the camera attached to the eye piece of the scope. The frame was then disconnected and the operation completed as usual. This initial experience was invaluable in assessing various points in the procedure. The principal finding was that the attachment mechanism of the frame was insufficiently secure and that some form of support other than the operating table would be required. Numerous other adjustments and refinements were also required. Once these were made several further patients were treated successfully in this 'semi-manual manner'.

It was at about this time that the closure of the Shaftesbury Hospital and the move to the Middlesex Hospital occurred. The whole scheme came to a halt. As described above my venue of operation had ultimately been transferred to Guy's Hospital. I had no NHS junior staff to work with on the problem and it still seemed doomed to abeyance.

At this awkward time I had working with me in my private practice a young Indian surgeon to whom I mentioned the project. Senthil Nathan. He was very intrigued when I explained the situation. Meanwhile, the Robotics Department at Imperial College had continued on their own with the project and had developed a miniature ultrasonic scanner mounted on a small probe that could be passed down the endoscope sheath and so arranged to scan the prostate at 2.0 mm intervals as it was mechanically withdrawn down the sheath by a further electric motor. These images were linked to a computer which was programmed to store the delineated measured anatomy of the prostate and project it as a two-dimensional representation on a visual display unit [Fig. 29.4]. Then by using a light pen it was possible to indicate accurately by drawing on the screen the area of prostatic tissue that was required to be removed. This information was stored on the computer. The ultrasound probe was next removed and a vaporising diathermy loop mounted on a conventional resectoscope was substituted. The computer was activated and controlled the three electric motors that were mounted on the ring to produce the cutting movements dictated by the scan as indicated above. This all worked quite well in the laboratory. Senthil picked up the problem with enthusiasm and with the Robotics department at Imperial College developed a secure mounting for the ring — separate from the operating table in the nature of an electronically controlled gantry on which the ring was mounted and which when not activated allowed the ring to be easily moved in any direction and allow the correct alignment of the endoscope in the

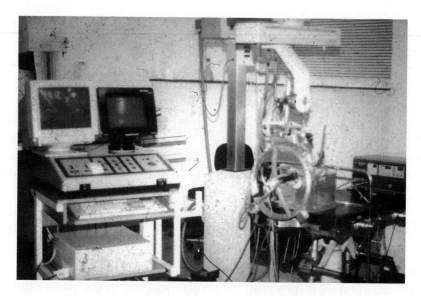

Fig. 29.4.   Instrument set-up in laboratory, Imperial College.

urethra of the patient much easier to achieve. The gantry was then activated electrically and controlled by foot pedal which when pressed solidly locked the gantry and frame so that there could be no movement of the instrument from its optimum position. All this preliminary work was carried out in the laboratory [Fig. 29.4].

Finally, it was decided that the instrument was fit for a clinical trial and under permission from Guy's we transferred the whole apparatus from Imperial College to the operating theatre there [Figs. 29.5–29.7]. We had contacted a suitable patient and once again explained the whole procedure to him as to what we were trying to achieve i.e. a very accurate means of treating his problem using a new robot with of course the proviso that we would immediately revert to a standard surgical manoeuvre if all was not completely satisfactory.

One of the previous problems with the standard resectoscope diathermy cutting loop was the difficulty of dealing with the excised 'prostatic chips' that it produced and which we had originally tried to avoid when attempting to develop the high speed drilling instrument many years before. Since that time, various companies had produced a range of resectoscopes using a new type of diathermy

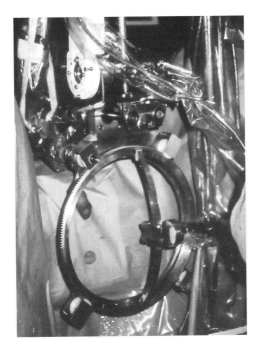

Fig. 29.5. Instrument set-up in theatre, Guy's Hospital.

current which instead of cutting the prostate vaporised it to a fine powdering of tissue which could easily be flushed out of the bladder. We had previously used this vaporising method successfully on a number of patients for conventional transurethral operation and had already published a paper on this method. We now found that this was ideal for the Probot as there were no 'chips' to obstruct the in and out movements of the diathermy electrode.

So, the anxious day arrived to try out this apparatus. The patient was anaesthetised. The endoscope was passed into his urethra and the frame suspended from the gantry, aligned with the endoscope sheath and all locked into place. The ultrasonic probe was passed down the sheath and the computer was started and the scanning completed. The 'to be resected area' was marked out on the VDU screen with a light pen [Fig. 29.8]. The scanning probe was removed, and the diathermy probe and telescope were passed. The irrigation was initiated, the diathermy connected, the camera

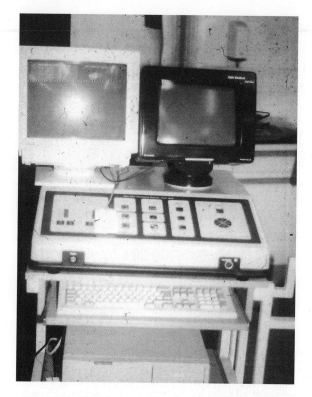

Fig. 29.6.   Master control desk of probot.

attached and the prostate visualised. We all stood waiting for the guillotine to fall as the start button was pushed. The whole apparatus came to life, the endoscope moved in and out, around the frame and across the diameter strut on the ring and we watched on the VDU as the diathermy electrode gradually vaporised the prostate, from the bladder neck to verumontanium. There was very little bleeding. Finally on completion everyone cheered, this being the second time that I had experienced such exuberance in the operating theatre since the first percutaneous stone removal! This was the very first time in the world that a robot had completely and autonomously operated on a patient without an operator moving a finger! Nearly, all other instruments still at the present time of writing, 2016, have been so-called 'surgeon assist robots' and not totally

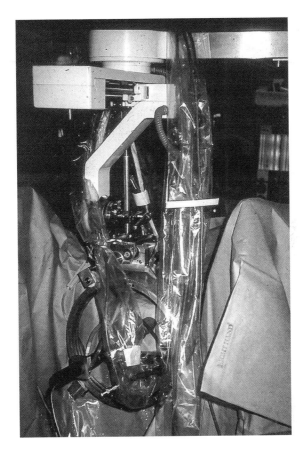

Fig. 29.7. Ready-to go probot in theatre, Guy's hospital.

freely acting without a guiding surgical hand being moved during the actual operation!

We had not had to use the large red emergency stop button on the apparatus and this was of course a complete vindication of the work of Professor Davies and his several colleagues at the Robotic Department at Imperial College.

At the end of the procedure, we took the resectoscope over manually, coagulated a few small bleeding vessels and the instrument was removed. The catheter was passed and the patient transferred to recovery. The duration of the procedure had been similar

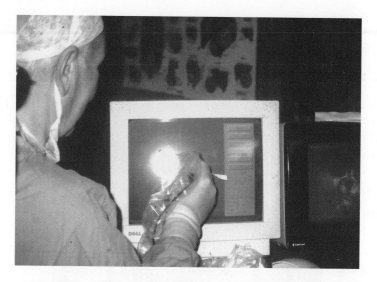

Fig. 29.8.   Drawing projected resection on screen with light pen.

to the hand held operation apart from a slightly longer setting up time. The end result was clinically perfectly satisfactory. We were all vastly encouraged by this and subsequently about 20 patients were successfully treated by either Senthil or myself with only minor modifications to the instrument as we proceeded. I found it quite a weird experience during an operation to sit with my arms folded watching the robot complete its work in April 1991.

Finally, it was interesting that as some patients in the ward who had had treatment by this method were saying 'I've had my operation done by the Robot'. Others were asking 'Please doctor can I have mine done by the Robot as well?' Such is the attraction of Science Fiction!

This was the culmination of much work by many persons. The major construction was obviously down to Professor Davies and his team but the part played by various members of the Institute of Urology was considerable starting with Malcolm Coptcoat, followed by Anthony Timoney and then Senthil Nathan.

The time then came for a meeting with the Robotics team and our own Medical side. I asked Brian Davies 'Where do we go from here?' he said 'The whole instrument wants re-engineering to make it more easily usable in an operating theatre.' 'How much will that cost?' I asked, conscious that we had done all our part of this work on research grant money. He said 'about £300–400,000.' Here, practicality set in. Would anyone be prepared to fund such an enterprise in the hope that this very complex piece of machinery could be brought into every day hospital use?

Commercially, the project did not make economic sense i.e. to do a costly operation that albeit was probably slightly more accurate but also one that could be done by a competent urologist did not make sense. Herewith, I learnt another of life's huge lessons. 'Do not stray into commercial waters about which one is ignorant and think things through to a sensible conclusion before embarking on a speculative and complex project'. It was, however, a world first in 1992 and clearly demonstrated how mechanics and robotics could be safely introduced into a clinical situation. This has been completely confirmed by the success of the da Vinci surgeon assist apparatus now in frequent clinical use. There is much more to come!

At this time, Andy Adam and I presented our design for a new interventional radiological and endoscopic suite at Guy's Hospital. We had to present our plans to the CEO of Guy's and St Thomas's. This person I had met before when he was CEO of St Peter's Hospital prior to its closure.

He listened to our plans for the specific area at Guy's and then told us it would not be possible to proceed as the area previously specified was now required for a cardiac facility and that our plan would be transferred to St Thomas's Hospital in three or four years. Same old story. It was then I finally gave up and retired to Private Practice.

Chapter 30

Postretirement from the NHS and Spreading the Word on Minimally Invasive Surgery

When I retired from the National Health Service in 1992, I continued with my private practice in Devonshire Place for two to three years and operated at the London Clinic and King Edward VII Hospital. I finally retired and I must here acknowledge with profound gratitude the tremendous help and back up that I received from many loyal secretaries. I have mentioned most in the narrative but I cannot fail to acknowledge the immense debt of gratitude I owe to my last loyal, honest and ever helpful PA Anneka Kelly, now Wright, who over a period of 20 years supported me unendingly and who has been dragged out of retirement to type this manuscript, she being the only person who can decode my appalling writing. My final operation at the London Clinic took place in 1998 [Fig. 30.1].

As time went on in the 1990s and stemming from the fact that I had written and talked about the benefits of Minimally Invasive Therapy, I was more and more frequently asked to travel to various parts of the country and of the world to spread the 'Heresy'. These visits took the form of either a single lecture or over two to three days as a so-called visiting Professorship. I was checking through my memory and roughly computed that these amounted to between 30–40 visits over about ten years. They were for me of considerable

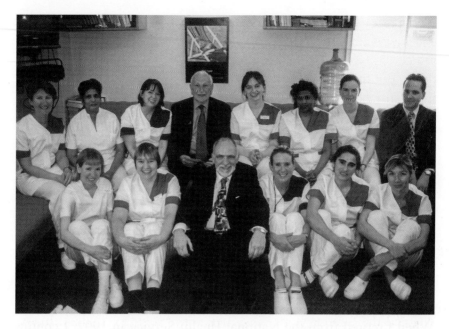

Fig. 30.1.   Last operation at the London clinic.

interest and one made many more lasting friendships. It is obviously impossible to detail them all but it is probably worth mentioning a few outstanding ones that remain in my consciousness for various reasons — some quite amusing.

In 1993, I was awarded the Cecil Joll prize of the Royal College of Surgeons of England for contributions to the 'Minimally Invasive Treatment' of renal disease. This was coupled with giving a talk on my work with MIT to an assembly of all grades and specialities of surgeons at the college. As usual, I tried to project my own experiences and aired my prejudices. I could feel from the audience reaction that what I had to say was not particularly appreciated by some although I did receive quite a few supportive remarks afterwards. One of which was 'Not bad old chap, but I don't think half of them understood or appreciated what you were saying' comes to mind but I hope that I may have indicated that there was perhaps an increasingly urgent need to review the accepted modes of instruction for young surgeons at that time.

At other venues, it was quite obvious that the reaction of the audiences was ambivalent. People do not like being told that what they are currently doing is possibly not the best way to go about something. But thankfully in recent years many practical courses involving instruction in MIT type procedures at the College of Surgeons and other University venues have emerged.

From Urological gatherings the reception was usually good, possibly because as a professional group we were much more familiar with the use of endoscopes and their possibilities.

From other specialities, acceptance appeared more slowly. In Tubingen in Germany, I met and formed another lifelong friendship with Professor Gerhardt Buess a colorectal surgeon who had developed a purely endoscopic method of selectively treating malignant lesions of the rectum and lower sigmoid colon by endoscopic intraluminal resection. Procedures were performed trans-anally with a large diameter endoscopic sheath passed through the anus that enabled the tumour to be identified. The rectum was then dilated and secondary instruments were passed down multiple operating channels in the primary instrument so that he could meticulously excise the tumour together with the whole thickness of the bowel wall and repair it. By using this method for some patients, he removed the need for what I always regarded as one of the most barbaric operations in the whole surgical repertoire, 'abdominoperineal resection,' i.e. the total excision of the whole rectum and anal sphincters plus the establishment of a colostomy for the treatment of a local lesion in the rectum thereby consigning the patient to years of discomfort, embarrassment and inconvenience and possible urinary incontinence. His results were equal to those reported for the previous open procedures for suitable lesions and the reaction of his colleagues to his manoeuvre were similar to those which I had experienced. We became friends, frequently agreed and occasionally disagreed with each other over some details but he joined me as the Deputy Editor of the *SMIT Journal* and was extremely helpful in dealing with some of the publishers and contributors. He unfortunately died in 2012, but has left a tremendous legacy in his speciality. It is of interest to note that in 1993 when I mentioned this new procedure to colleagues in Colo-rectal surgery in London no one had heard of it!

In 1993 and before in Scandinavia especially in Sweden, I gave a number of talks and actually ran courses in percutaneous stone surgery at the University of Gothenburg with Michael Kellet and Ron Miller. Again, I made another very fond friend in Professor Silas Petterson, Senior Urologist, with whom I still keep in close contact. He in fact promoted the fact that I was conferred with the honorary degree of Dr of Medicine in The University of Gothenburg in 1994.

In Copenhagen, I was also presented with the Rovsing Medal of the Danish Surgical Society after giving a lecture on MIT.

At home in 1993, I was asked to give a talk to the Royal Society of Radiologists in view of my writings in which I constantly pointed out the vital importance of the combination of Radiologists with Surgeons in a number of the new interventional procedures that were being introduced. I could not have managed what we were trying to achieve in urology without the close cooperation of my friend and colleague, Mike Kellett. I gave the lecture and was awarded the Cook Medal of the Royal Society of Radiologists.

Also in 1993, the Royal Society of Radiologists conferred their Honorary Fellowship of the Society on me the FRCR.

Even more surprising was that in the same month I received the news that the Royal College of Physicians of London had conferred their Honorary Fellowship on me the FRCP — both awards being a little unusual for a surgeon. Someone must have appreciated the kernel of the message that I was trying to get across. "Don't damage people to perform an elective operation"!

With Professor Andy Adam, my Radiological colleague, I attended the annual meeting of the Western Angiographic Society in Portland, OR, USA. This was held in the Hospital that the famous Radiologist Professor Seldinger had first performed his now standard technique for the introduction of specially designed catheters into the arterial circulation of either leg or arm as a preparation for

the diagnosis and treatment of various forms of disease of the vascular system by angioplasty particularly those of the coronary arteries but also of other peripheral vessels. The Professor was still very active.

This meeting was interesting because there were about 200 plus Interventional Radiologists being addressed by a Surgeon. I gave a talk on how we had very successfully combined with our radiological colleagues to perform PCN etc. in the UK and emphasised there should be many more similar collaborations. To my surprise, I was quite aggressively attacked by some of the delegates, the message being — 'We don't want surgeons moving into our area of expertise as we are very rapidly going to oust surgeons from this field completely.' They would hardly listen to my explanations of collaboration and I very much had the impression that their anger had a significant financial basis. A totally new experience for me being used to UK NHS thinking.

Other interesting invitations were received. One of these was to visit the Department of Bioengineering at the Cleveland Clinic, USA from a Professor Fred Cornhill, Head of Department. It emerged later that he had read my article in the *British Medical Journal* and said 'We must invite this odd man to come and talk to us about his peculiar ideas.'

I duly turned up, gave a talk which went down all right and was then invited to come back again and give it to a larger audience the following year. After my second visit, I then received an invitation from the American Society of Bioengineering to give the Plenary address to the Annual Meeting of the Society also being held that particular year in Cleveland. The audience was quite receptive and a copy of the Editorial in their Journal of 1998 can explain the reception better than I can and also illuminate what I was expounding but which was not always well received by older surgeons both in Europe and the USA. The Bioengineers, however, seemed to like it which encouraged me considerably and the Editorial in the *Bioengineering Journal* was also encouraging and amusing here reproduced below.

When Less Is More: Minimally Invasive Therapies Herald Maximally Influential Changes

Medical Device & Diagnostic Industry
Magazine, November 1, 1998

Among the most enduring images of modern medicine is that of the lone surgeon—the last line of defense—standing fast against disease and death with an armament of art, science, and cold steel. What, then, could provoke a distinguished member of this heroic band to depict his fellow practitioners as "Neanderthals . . . a species that certainly should become extinct in the next 20 years"? And why would such a heretic be the featured speaker at a gathering of biomedical engineers?

John E.A. Wickham, senior research fellow and surgeon at Guy's Hospital in London, is credited with coining the term "minimally invasive surgery" and with organizing the first MIS department, set up at the University of London's Institute of Urology in 1986. In his plenary address during the recent annual meeting of the Biomedical Engineering Society, held in Cleveland, Wickham proposed a scenario for the future of minimally invasive therapies that, if accurate, holds profound implications not only for health-care providers but for the device industry as well.

In brief, Wickham predicts that the traditional domains of the "open" surgeon will be rapidly taken over by teams of endoscopists and interventional radiologists, working closely with bioengineers and instrument manufacturers. These changes would apply to most current surgical specialties, encompassing urologic, obstetric/gynecologic, gastrointestinal, orthopedic, neurologic, cardiothoracic, and vascular procedures. The fact that minimally invasive operative methods are becoming more common is neither new nor surprising, given that the techniques can often reduce patient morbidity and save money compared with standard treatments.

But Wickham foresees a more extensive transformation resulting from the wide-scale adoption of minimally invasive therapies. Demands for new technology will include the need for more sophisticated equipment, ranging from miniaturized scopes to advanced tissue-manipulation and tissue-lesioning tools, active and diagnostic robotics, and next-generation imaging devices and optics. Anesthesia practices will follow trends in surgery, with more emphasis on peripheral nerve blocks and the development of "on/off," reverse-potential blocks. Operating suites and radiology rooms will have to be reengineered to accommodate new equipment, personnel, patient-transport systems, and work-flow patterns. Common ailments involving diverse organ groups will be treated at peripheral facilities staffed by "general" endoscopic surgeons and interventional radiologists, with the more complicated procedures done at regional centers by "intensivists" in the same disciplines.

How quickly these events are realized will largely depend, says Wickham, on "whether the diffusion of new technology is to be guided by physicians or by politicians." If health-care policy does not become more supportive of technological innovation, Wickham fears that the physician's "flexible, discretionary judgement necessary for patient well-being" will continue to be compromised by government regulation and market forces intent on preserving the status quo. He quotes J. S. Mill, who found that "the despotism of custom is everywhere the standing hindrance to human achievement." It might even keep some of the smarter Neanderthals standing around the tables a few extra years.

Promoting innovative technology is also the focus of the second annual Medical Design Excellence Awards, sponsored by *MDDI*'s publisher Canon Communications. I want to remind our readers that the deadline to submit entries for the competition is February 8, 1999. Information on how to achieve recognition for the product(s) of your inspiration can be found at www.devicelink.com/awards.

Jon Katz

Incidentally, I was told later that the Department of Urology at the Cleveland Clinic was somewhat annoyed that I had been in the Establishment and they did not know I was there because they felt that my presentation should have been given under their auspices. You can't please everyone as I commonly found out!

A few other remembrances of visiting professorships:

In Houston having given a talk I was presented with a rather beautiful Stetson hat as a reminder of Texas. Unfortunately, this was about four sizes too large and as I was crowned with this masterpiece it came down completely over my head so I could neither hear nor see. Much laughter and cheers.

In Philadelphia being driven from hotel to hospital my driver suddenly slowed to less than walking pace for about half a mile. I asked why he was going so slowly. He said "In this area the local trick is to rush out in front of an auto and pretend to have been run over. The driver is then sued. At this speed, no one comes to any harm!" We got there and the presentation appeared well received.

In Lexington, KY to do a demonstration percutaneous nephrolithotomy. Into the operating theatre with a 20-stone patient on the table! 'Where is the radiologist to do the tracking?' 'There is no one who can do it. We thought you were automatous.' Initial panic and I tried to remember how Michael Kellett performed. With great pot luck, I managed to needle the kidney and remove the stone. Another hypertensive episode!

In New York installed in the United Nations Plaza Hotel on the 23rd floor. At about 8.00 pm retired to bed after transatlantic flight. 8.30 pm knock on the door — young lady offering her services. Declined. 9.00 pm fire alarm goes off. Look out of window and rather startled to see fire trucks and ambulances assembled 22 floors below. Managed to get out to the ground floor down 23 flights of steps in pyjamas with the fire alarm going constantly because the lifts were shut off. False alarm set off by the aforementioned young lady who had triggered the alarm by forcing her way through a fire door.

Back to bed 10.00 pm. Phone call 'very urgent package in reception'. Dressed and got to reception. The package was four copies of a recent book that I had edited — sent by the publishers in case I wanted to introduce it after my following day lecture, back to bed at 11.00 pm. Fretful sleep, up early to the hospital. 10.00 am — gave lecture with much discussion at New York University Hospital, then taken to lunch and Broadway to see a show back to hotel then to the airport — total collapse! It is a hard peripheral life being a surgeon! Alternatively, keep your mouth shut.

En route from Ancona initially where I had been lecturing to Padua to give another talk. Stopped at a rather smart hotel on the coast. Had dinner. 12.00 midnight — considerable intestinal commotion. I had some antibiotics in the car outside. As I snuck across the foyer in my pyjamas the main door opened to reveal six persons in immaculate evening dress. Stood to one side to let them pass looking like a refugee from a down and out encampment. *'Bueno notte signor'* with much sniggering! One must always keep up appearances no matter the emergency!

Back in the UK in 1994, I was pursuing my usual line of thinking and wrote an updating article for the *British Medical Journal*. Again, I received a number of slightly more encouraging remarks.

Another invitation was to give a talk at Massachusetts General Hospital USA in the 'Ether Dome', the original operating theatre where in 1846 Morton gave the first general anaesthetic to a patient in public and an operation was carried out without needing patient restraint. It was a great honour to speak in this hallowed venue which had seen the inauguration of practically the greatest advance in surgical progress which had ever been experienced.

From time to time, it was interesting to hear the old argument of Minimally Invasive versus Minimal Access Surgery being used. Some people did not seem to grasp the basic concept that not damaging tissue wherever possible was paramount — not just reducing the access of entry. Things have moved on a little since 1994.

Thanks to Ron Miller's and John Fitzpatrick's help, we were able to progress the *Journal of Minimally Invasive Therapy* and also give sustaining secretarial help between the annual conference and with the organisation of the Society Meetings at many venues. Here our Secretary, Fay Harrison, was indefatigable and irreplaceable.

After the first London meeting, further gatherings took place at many venues both in the UK and abroad. See brochure title pages for Berlin and Kyoto (Appendix 3).

London in 1989
Vienna in 1990
Boston, USA in 1991
Dublin in 1992
Orlando, USA in 1993
Berlin in 1994
Portland, USA in 1995
Milan in 1996
Kyoto in 1997
and London in 1998.

Since that time, further annual meetings have continued and taken place all over Europe and the Far East. For instance, in 2014, the 26th meeting took place in Shanghai in China. It is of interest to note that no additional gatherings have taken place in the USA since 1999 — why, I don't know.

Those meetings that were locally organised in each country by numerous people were as far as I could determine well received and informative and we had attendance levels of about 400 delegates at each. The organisers were many and among the most prominent were John Fitzpatrick in Dublin, Bruce McLucas in Boston and Gehardt Buess in Berlin.

In the UK Ron Miller, Malcolm Coptcoat, Michael Kellett and Andy Adam gave a vast amount of help without which we would never have kept going. It is sad to observe however over the succeeding 25-year period how the innovative clinical contribution from the UK was gradually being eroded possibly by the increased regulatory restrictions being placed on UK clinicians. Time for active clinical research was being subtly reduced because of the introduction of time restrictions and targets which still continue today. Most activity now emanates from the USA, Germany and the Far East, Japan and lately China.

I was fortunate that I was able to control my own activities and continued as the Honorary Life President of the Society with each annual event being organised by a local Chairman which still continues. Many of the surgical procedures that have now become routine were first aired at the Society meetings and were received with interest and some with scepticism.

By 1997, it was time to withdraw from my commitments to the Society and hand over the Secretarial arrangements. The last meeting I was involved in organising was in London in 1998 and was my farewell to the Society. For this meeting, we had to move the Secretarial arrangements to my office in Devonshire Place because of the geographical difficulties of moving to and from the central London hotel selected for its amenities and accommodation for delegates and we vacated our office from Guy's Hospital for this meeting. I was much relieved to give up the Editorial responsibility for the Journal which was assumed by Professor Buess.

A London member of the Society volunteered to take over and assume the organisational and editorial aspects of the Society's activities and as Fay also wished to retire it was suggested that the office and archives should be moved to this other major London Teaching Hospital. This was done and we relaxed a little.

After a few months nothing much seemed to happen and there appeared to be no evidence of preparations for the next annual meeting. Colleagues from abroad, particularly in Germany, were beginning to agitate and question me as to what was happening. I was not able to give them any information and referred them to the person who had assumed responsibility. Nothing seemed forthcoming and finally colleagues in Germany were so dismayed that one weekend they arrived in London with a transit van, collected the necessary documentation and took the whole archives of the Society back to Germany and fired everything up again. Thus, SMIT became a German organisation administered from Neiderhausen and continues to prosper.

Once again it confirmed to me that the UK neither politically nor scientifically had little use for such an entity! Advances in surgery and medicine are initiated by enthusiastic scientists and clinicians and not by politicians and managerial theorists who have effectively curtailed some medical innovation in this country. Perhaps, it is not considered important that any innovation should necessarily be originated in the UK?

It would seem that by political and administrative decree, it has been decided that the health service is purely what it is designated 'a service' and scientific innovation will be discouraged and advances in medicine will be adopted as necessary from countries abroad who still have the finance and are free to pursue and develop new therapies e.g. lithotripters from Germany, da Vinci's from the USA.

In 2008, I was elected an Honorary Fellow of the Royal Society of Medicine — amazing! I had been an ordinary paying Fellow since the 1970s. The honour was extremely nice to receive but I still have to pay for the privilege!

Chapter 31

Syclix — Now What Was
I to do With My Time?

Another small experimental programme was unwisely started by myself at the point of retirement in 1992 when my Accountant asked me how I was going to spend my time.

For about 10 years, I had had the idea that it would be interesting to develop a small facility for producing innovative surgical instrumentation. What I had in mind was for a range of delicate hand held instruments for delicate surgery. This would obviously require supportive finance and the Accountant suggested a person who we both knew and who had incidentally been a patient of mine and might be interested in investing in such a scheme.

We arranged a meeting and I explained my ideas and the friend was happy to join in and finance such a project on a 51%–49% share basis. I was very happy with this and set to work on a scheme which for various reasons extended over a 13-year period and the company was called Syclix.

My basic idea was to develop delicate instruments with an entirely new mechanism for holding in the hand but with the movements of the jaws, either forceps or scissors, currently being powered by a scissor type of ring grip being replaced by a compression pad that could be easily squeezed by finger pressure and arranged so that this could be produced on the pad at any angle of 360 degrees and transferred to a mechanical shaft to activate the jaws. The whole instrument could be rotated by finger movement only and not by wrist or elbow.

This effect would enable the jaws to be powered in any orientation of the shaft of the instrument unlike that produced by ring grips which frequently require the fingers to be released from the rings and then often re-inserted in a different position with difficulty at an inconvenient time in an operative procedure.

I knew an industrial designer with whom I had worked before and put the plan to him and we agreed to proceed. Here is where I made another of my huge lifestyle mistakes. Do *NOT* venture into territory of which one is not fully informed and for which one is not trained i.e. trying to compete with established companies doing this type of business and especially not produce instrumentation that you may personally consider invaluable but which have not been requested by other colleagues and may afford competition to manufacturers!

The designer over a number of months produced prototype instruments which I said I would like to appear and be held in the hand like a Mont Blanc writing pen, would be as comfortable to use and which would make any number of operative manoeuvres less acrobatic.

The next step was to investigate the patent possibilities of the device. Not un-expectantly, patents had already been filed for devices along the same lines. The powering mechanisms were all different but with considerable effort it became possible to navigate around these claims and finally register our own design. This of course took considerable time, ingenuity and a substantial amount of investment.

The next step involved various decisions.

(1) Disposable or reusable — at this time, there was much discussion on the transmission of the bovine encephalopathy virus on reusable surgical instruments and I had already published two submitted papers from Germany in the *SMIT Journal* indicating the impossibility of completely cleaning and re-sterilising reusable instruments which were constructed with a shaft and pull rod design. The decision was therefore to go for a disposable range. This decision predicated that the bulk of each instrument should be plastic, disposable metal being far too expensive to consider.

So, the next step was to relate to plastic manufacturers and the first firm we approached produced moulds for instruments that turned out to be too crude. So onto another company who finally produced an acceptable device. There was much discussion on biocompatibility of various plastics which was finally solved by this second Company.

(2) The regulatory aspects of the project needed to be considered with quality control companies consulted together with company insurance etc. and how to gain a CE marking to permit marketing in Europe and FDA approved in the USA.

As one can imagine, all these considerations took up an interminable amount of time and a not inconsiderable amount of financial input. It became obvious that there was a need to employ some sort of whole time business manager who had experience of this type of situation and a suitable person was selected again at more expense. An office and secretary followed. The finance department was by now getting a little anxious and I was obviously becoming more out of my depth and expertise.

(3) Finally, suitable instrumentation was produced after all the above hurdles had been surmounted [Figs. 31.1 and 3.12].

In a 'catch 22' situation, it was impossible to evaluate the instruments until they were fully developed and available in a form suitable for clinical use. So, the next step was to test the interest of colleagues who could actually use and handle the instruments in the operating theatre when completed. We submitted them to a number of surgeons who produced almost the same assessment. 'We like them very much but we need a little more power for closure of the jaws.' A diathermy facility on some instruments was desired and a jaw locking mechanism on others. We therefore produced hand machined prototypes of all these modifications to satisfy these demands! One should bear in mind that each instrument was made up of about ten moulded parts. Each mould was individually machined and cost about £5000–£7000 to produce. To change even minor points in construction would be expensive. Things and timings were getting out of hand and there had been a considerable of financial outlay.

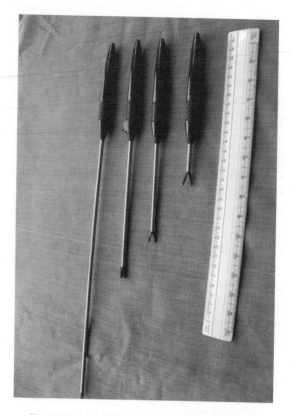

Fig. 31.1. Syclix Instruments, variable lengths.

We now made the decision to set up a small marketing facility to test purchaser interest but then disaster struck. Finance had been supplied in considerable amounts over an 8–10-year period and there was increasing reluctance to spend the necessary amount of equity to produce and supply the modifications requested.

Secondly and far more importantly, our backing friend had developed a severe mental illness which incapacitated him so badly that he was unable to be involved in any business decisions. The management of his affairs was transferred to a Trust, the Chairman of which decided that they no longer wished to support any commercial project of this nature. We were not the only company in the backing group so affected.

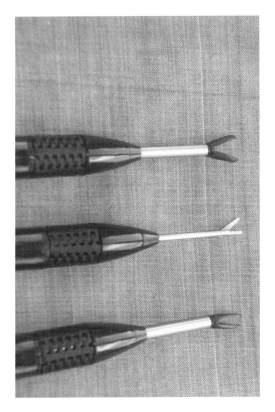

Fig. 31.2.   Syclix Instruments, detail of jaws.

Despite numerous discussions and suggestions, the project passed into abeyance and despite interest expressed by other instrument manufacturers no agreements could be reached because of the accumulated investment costs already incurred and the insistence of the trustees that these should be amortized before making any further instrumentation or arrangements.

To repeat my previous warning — Firstly, do not undertake large projects of things of which you only have a one-sided knowledge or large operations for which you are too ill-informed to undertake. 'A houseman doing an aortic resection!' Also, do not undertake projects as a *part-time hobby* of something that requires 24/7 full time attention.

Secondly, the fact that because one felt personally that these instruments were surgically advantageous did not necessarily chime with the opinions of those who were quite happy with what they were already using and on which they had been trained.

Finally having discussed the problems with some of my friends in the instrument business they were all surprised that we had got so far on a relatively small outlay — the quoted amount that they would have laid out on such a project would have been in the order of 5 million pounds or more.

The instruments were stored in a warehouse but have now in 2016 been destroyed. The moulds could possibly be reactivated if someone was prepared to act swiftly.

So plans for a retirement interest hit the buffers despite all these long years of effort! It may be that someone may be interested in reviving this project. All the bits are there and with minor modification and further capital I still feel that such instrumentation could be useful. Also, in this period, I was working at Guy's when other matters of interest arose. In view of our work with the Probot, I was invited to come and address a number of meetings on Robotic surgery as we truly had been the first group in the world to use such an instrument in the clinical situation.

While travelling in the USA I had the opportunity to visit the facility in Santa Barbara in California to talk with the principal designers at the company that were at the time developing the concepts and prototypes of what was to become the Leonardo da Vinci instrument. It was obvious that this was going to succeed and become the valuable piece of equipment that is now so well appreciated and is taking endoscopic surgery to another level. This situation reminded me very much of the early days of the Dornier Lithotripter.

The da Vinci surgeon assist instrument now well established in a number of hospitals has clearly indicated one of the several ways in which interventional medicine should be progressing. I think the most important attributes of this instrument are the magnification of the target area of the operation. Secondly, the operator's hands are moved away from the operative area and visual tremor is almost eliminated by computer control leading again to a very marked increase in precision.

It always amazed me that in the 21st century surgeons continued to stand swaying at a work bench like a kitchen table with the operative target two to three feet away from them. The need to stand for long periods and to keep adjusting one's posture leads to decreased stability and manual inaccuracy. This was one reason I had very early on in my career arranged that as far as possible when I was performing surgery I should be able for both visual and manual reasons, to sit down and be as close as possible to the area of action. The da Vinci does all this splendidly. Certainly, it is complex but not difficult to learn and it's not beyond the capabilities of most surgeons to achieve competence. It was when I tried my remaining expertise on a da Vinci simulator that I was delighted to find how easy it was to master the mechanism. It was the one time that I felt that I would love to return to clinical medicine and utilise it. It was the culmination of many of the desiderata that I wished had been available when I was working! This and similar robotic machinery I am sure is the way forward in much interventional medicine and reiterates the same old situation — "Expensive machinery initially difficult to learn to use = very slow take up especially in the NHS" which returns me to the point mentioned previously that the increasing costs of technology will exponentially continue to make significant demands on funding.

Who at which point in the development of a new technique or medication which is successful coupled with patient demand will decide the cut-off point to NHS additional funding? In whose interest is it to keep many old people alive and functioning by means of these elegant machines. I am glad that I will not be around to have to make this increasingly important decision which seems to becoming more philosophical than purely clinical.

No matter what eventuates and what demands are made on healthcare interventional therapy is inexorably destined to become more visually focussed, more targeted, more accurate, less traumatic, more expensive but less dreaded by patients. It may well be that gradually the physicians may solve many of the problems now requiring mechanical intervention and surgery in various areas will wither!

So, my surgical experience was stimulated by the need to embrace an entirely different Mode of activity. I feel that I was very privileged to have been part of this change over point from butchery to mechanistic expertise. The opportunities for the application of more complex robotic apparatus are unlimited. I can visualise malignant material in any organ being much more accurately delineated by advanced imaging then being removed by robotic machinery with an accuracy that will be far more precise than that which could possibly be achieved by the human hand. What an exciting prospect! for the Clinician, what a nightmare for the provider of funding be it Government or Individual!

Chapter 32

The Answers to the Initial Three Questions

I hope by now I have answered the primary questions?

So what does all this amount to? Have the three questions been thoroughly addressed?

(1) How did you become a surgeon? Has been described exhaustively at the various stages in the training process and I can add no more.
(2) Why did you become a surgeon — fortuitously and because of the scientific interest and enjoyment of the clinical process.
(3) The third question — what is it like to be a surgeon? Is obviously more complex with many unsuspected 'add-ons', many not strictly clinical.

One feature that I have not emphasised in this description is the psychological wear and tear that you were subjected to as one was moved up the complexity scale of the work. Each step involved another bout of differing anxieties as to whether or not one could cope with the mechanics of the advancement. Another peripheral worry occurred occasionally when actively performing an operation; was it entirely for the patient's benefit? Had you improved the situation, had you harmed them or were you just enjoying doing surgery because you could? One very important decision point I learnt from Alec Badenoch was when *not* to operate. It is all too easy to proceed to something which has little benefit for the patient.

Waiting day by day as to the outcome of a procedure was ever evident and wondering if everything would work out correctly was an ambient form of anxiety and one which never went away even after many years in the business. The postoperative morning round was occasionally tinged with mild apprehension. At least that is what I experienced for once embarked on surgery as a career one was consistently involved in some way or other with little let up. Looking back over this long period I did not at the time come to fully appreciate the vulnerable situation in which one was placed. I cannot think of many professions where one is fully licensed to significantly damage another human albeit being with good intent. One can of course go into all this in a cavalier fashion, picking up a knife and rendering a wound in a person's body all within the permitted law. I did not appreciate what a fantastic amount of trust a patient invests in the relationship with and judgement of his or her surgical manipulator and this has occasionally given me much cause for thought. It is a hard task to work consistently so as to fulfil this remit as there can *never* be any margin for serious error, which if made, can be catastrophic for all concerned. I am sure it is inevitable that many surgeons like myself carry a varying degree of guilt over some situations that could in retrospect have been better handled.

To this extent, this is what you take on when you decide to be a surgeon. It is really not a job for the faint hearted and no one pointed this out to me when I first started on the long trail. Maintaining a degree of humanity in all this I found difficult. One inevitably becomes a very full time operating technician and with the rapidity of turnover now demanded it becomes very difficult to establish any direct human relationship between patient and surgeon. I think my most genuine regret is that I did not spare more time with the patients as a true doctor and not so much as a technician. Pressure of work was the excuse but in retrospect this cannot be valid and if I was going through this again I know I would wish to spend more time listening and talking to a patient and try harder to relieve anxiety despite the pressure to achieve numbers and throughput. You can have a profession or a Job. The Public must choose.

Chapter 33

The National Health Service and its Impact on Medical Ethics

Over a 40-year period many associated changes occurred in medical practice apart from the developments in operative surgery described above and it is obviously impossible for one observer to itemise and comment on the multiplicity of various events that took place in this period. I can only report on a few of the changes that I personally experienced.

The Ethical Changes in Medicine and Nursing

As E. M. Forster observed in 1940 'The more highly public life is organised the lower it's morality sinks.' Unfortunately, one cannot but agree. This is evidenced within the National Health Service by the scandals being revealed in the daily press detailing the lack of compassion and care being demonstrated in our regulated hospitals by some of the medical and nursing staff. I cannot believe that this behaviour could have occurred at St Bartholomew's Hospital in the century before 1948 and even for a few years after. The Matron and the Governors would have soon extruded the culprits. What went on in hospitals in other parts of the country has not been recorded in so much detail as that which occurred in the London Teaching Hospitals. Peripheral hospitals did not seem to have undergone the same detailed scrutiny but as I recall were always much appreciated and respected by their local communities and the Nursing processes all seemed based on the teachings of the major Hospitals in the Capital and the larger Cities.

In a civilised society, there is surely no excuse for this terrible behaviour! These events are now being blamed on the increasing pressures caused by the number of ageing persons requiring hospital treatment, the insufficiency of medical and nursing staff on the ground, the rapid development of increasingly complex therapeutic procedures and finally the lack of finance that despite regular increments has now reached a crisis point. I would suggest another more important cause for these deficiencies — Abysmal management!

To relieve these problems the immediately suggested answer is for more financial input which is unlikely to be forthcoming in adequate quantity in the present difficult economic climate. Despite such measures I cannot see how one can possibly rewind the clock and reproduce the ethos that was displayed by doctors and nurses when the Health Service was inaugurated. They were the engine that drove the whole machine forward when I started my career. People have changed, society has radically changed and the altruism and goodwill of those entering the professions is very quickly curtailed and modified by the nature of the management structure as now developed.

Forty years ago, Doctors and Nurses were independent professionals of status deriving from their prolonged periods of training and academic education. Unfortunately, they have now been relegated to minor participants in an impersonal managerial machine with many unintended consequences.

My first experience of the intervention of modern management was in the 1970s when I became a Consultant. All seemed well organised and functioned smoothly. The system at Barts as I understood it at that time consisted of a number of clinical advisory committees made up of doctors and nurses who indicated their requirements to a lay Board of Governors. These appeared to accede to most requests. 'If that is what the doctors and nurses think is necessary for the patients we will if possible try to provide the required facilities.' This was within the constraints of a voluntary system of finance which encouraged a degree of parsimony and self-discipline in the clinical staff for the good functioning of the hospital, an attitude now absent due to the central nature of government funding!

The *small* number of paid administrators at the time followed the directions of the Governors and it was my experience that these persons were wise and reasonable. If one had cause to consult with them on any topic they were consistently helpful and came up with sensible responses and solutions to the clinical requirements of the medical and nursing staff. There was never any feeling of direction or coercion.

A flashing red warning light first occurred when it was suggested that I attend a course in management at the Kings Fund Organisation in Bayswater, London.

This was a two week assembly which comprised around 12 newly appointed Consultants in various specialities from hospitals all over the country. We were all of an age, late 30s, early 40s, and were then lectured to by a series of young persons who appeared to have just left school or university.

Various topics were discussed, some useful, some embarrassingly obvious but the crunch came on the last day when we were invited to discuss 'How can Management Discipline the Consultant Staff?' I was not aware that Consultants at this time were particularly in need of discipline but were regarded as responsible adults going about their professional duties in their hard won new appointments and working for the benefit of their patients.

This was a warning sign of coming events which I tended to ignore.

The second worrying event occurred at my first Consultant Medical Committee in Barts when one of our colleagues said 'I think you should all consider this document.' This was a copy of McKinsey and Company's report on the recommended management programme for the Oxford region of the NHS.

The essence was revealed by a flow chart of the proposed system. As I recall, this showed at the top a CEO, beneath, a layer of about four deputies, below this another larger level of even more managers and finally the crunch bottom line of fireman, ambulance man, cleaner, electrician, nurse, refuse collector, doctor, porter, painter, etc. It was clearly evident that doctors and nurses despite their professional expertise and extensive training were to be relegated to effector end organs of this vast system and were to be deployed as foot soldiers by this managerial officer elite. There was little evidence of any clinical input at the upper managerial levels of these new arrangements.

Coming events were certainly casting big shadows which as clinicians we tended to ignore and got on with our work of treating patients. While the looming of the MBA type of attitude now conveniently described as 'Medical Taylorism' (see Reference[*]) from the USA with its mantra of managerial control and centralisation of action into large complexes began to be apparent we took little notice. All surely seemed a negation of the primary medical process of the sympathetic treatment of one individual by another fully trained independent professional person being gradually taken over by the directions of a number of individuals on apparently lay committees. The remit of such committees seemed devoted to the measurement of the time taken by any clinical activity and to standardise all medical processes with a view to 'maximizing efficiency' and to define that there is only 'one best' way to perform any task which should then be strictly adhered to! There was to be no flexibility or independent activity.

It seems in retrospect that most medical staff at this time did not speak out and abdicated their *direct professional* responsibility for the welfare of their patients to this system and were thereby relegated to the position of a small cog of little influence in a proposed 'job' and would ultimately cease to be regarded as independent professionals. This was I believe the beginning of the erosion and loss of the professional medical ethic which in time has spread to a

---

[*]Reference Medical Taylorism — Hartzband P. Groopman J. *New England Journal of Medicine* Jan 14 (2016) 04-05.

number of younger persons now staffing some of our hospitals, vide The Stafford Hospital scandal and many more.

What was the Effect of this Newer Ethos on the Practice of Medicine?

I can only sensibly comment on the manner in which the nature of the Health Service changed in relation to surgery during the period when I was concerned but a brief look at what has happened to medicine in its entirety over this 40-year period is interesting. For one person to give a comprehensive appraisal and critique of such a complex system is not feasible and I can only point out some of the outstanding events which directly or indirectly impacted upon my professional life.

The National Health Service was introduced to this country in 1948 as an extremely bold and humane venture to alleviate some of the hardships felt by an extensive part of the population who had very poor access to health care and social security. It was a vast canvas and the changes in medical practice in general have been extensive over the years since its foundation.

1. General Practice

When I completed my primary training, most of my contemporaries were keen to embrace general practice as their life's work while a few of us were drawn into hospital medicine. We tended to look down on General Practitioners as somewhat second class citizens! I now feel totally embarrassed to recall this attribution. This is so horribly wrong as I discovered later and found out that General Practice as initially conceived is truly the 'heart' of Medical care and what 'Medicine' is all about. The General Practitioner is the primary physician upon whom the whole edifice of patient care is erected. It was they who could quickly define whether a patient was truly sick and needed active treatment or purely required friendly counselling or advice.

At this time in the later 1940s it was possible for the local doctor to personally know many patients on their list both ill or well and also as human beings with families of all age groups from newborns to geriatrics. Intimate knowledge of their family lives was usually the norm and although often excessively busy the doctor was nearly always available to be consulted as a clinician and a friend. In those days, it was not uncommon for a patient's General Practitioner to follow them to hospital and be available for discussions with the appropriate Consultants and a considerable liaison developed between the differing types of practice. The doctor knew the economic circumstances of the patients and altruism in the nature of recompense for many small services rendered was well recognised i.e. they treated these poorer patients and their families for free. Very importantly, they knew the patients face to face and not as a number of flickering bytes of information on a computer screen and actually made eye contact when being consulted.

In time, I witnessed a gradual erosion of this situation. I can't speak for General Practitioners but I was amazed at the conditions under which they functioned. Apart from working very long hours they were having to deal with a situation in most practices where it was not possible to obtain a simple blood test or X-ray result quickly and required patient referral to a General Hospital for such basic diagnostic requirements. As numbers of patients and complexity of diagnosis and therapy increased hospitals gradually became less able to deal with this influx of referred patients and the managerial engine moved into motion to sort all this out.

We all know now what has gradually eventuated. In what appears to be a frantic attempt to compensate for lack of clinical time and to shortage of General Practitioners with increasing patient numbers, bizarre managerial directives are now frequently being issued to doctors.

A few examples

(i) The instruction to limit consultation time to 10 minutes per symptom. More than one and the patient must come back for another '10 minutes' worth of attention at a later date. Such a system does not remotely allow time for a full discussion of a patient's problems, let alone examination. What a travesty and ignorance of the whole medical and diagnostic process! Can one imagine the reaction of a lawyer being told to investigate a complex legal problem and resolve it within 10 minutes!

I was taught what the famous Professor Osler of Oxford declaimed that 'One must always hear the patient out and the diagnosis will usually be revealed from the last remarks made by the patient on leaving the surgery'. Also, 'the first presenting symptom may not necessarily be related to the disorder suffered'. How very true!

Stop Press. Today 21st April 2016. The CEO of the NHS has announced that General Practitioners may now be given(sic) up to 30 minutes for a Consultation with a Patient. If the complaint is trivial the Patient may be sent off for a consultation with a Pharmacist or a Psychologist. At last, the 'General Practitioner is to be put back on his or her feet! One may well enquire who tripped them up in the first place? The CEO will, I am sure, be thanked for his kind permissive gift of another 20 minutes!'

(ii) More disastrous was the implementation of the politically inspired five day week and no weekend work contract introduced and which must take considerable responsibility for the shambolic situation that has now arisen. General Practice has now become a 9–5 'job' five days a week with no out of hours responsibility so that a physician should be fresh and not tired. Being a little fatigued as far as I was concerned was part of being a doctor but one coped! This vast gap in cover has produced a series of calamities made worse by the implementation of such mechanisms as the 111 telephone call system with its impersonal and interminable box ticking scenario with lay personnel or nurses on the line often unable to achieve a safe diagnosis, leading to the inevitable delayed referral to an A and E Department.

In another effort to achieve some cover is the employment of agency physicians at extraordinary expense and some of questionable professional standards, who often turn up several hours late and through lack of local knowledge and experience make significant mistakes in diagnosis and therapy. An even more alarming managerial directive to the South East Ambulance system covering Sussex, Surrey and part of Kent is also worthy of remark. This was recently instructed that when a true emergency had been identified by the 111 system and was one that required a 999 rapid response reaction, the management had decided that the response should be delayed because it might disturb the targeted response times of the 999 system.

Because of this ruling, patients may well have died! If this is correct, then a situation approaching a state of corporate manslaughter by this management system has surely been reached managerial decisions completely denying clinical necessity. Now the latest digital disaster waiting to happen is the computer consultation.

(iii) *The Computer Consultation*: It has now been decided that a computer consultation with a patient's General Practitioner can be carried out on line. A patient of say 80 years with indifferent IT skills may at last contact a doctor on screen. Firstly, is the patient conscious, and mentally competent? If so, a history may be obtained but what of the physical examination? Has the patient a fever, high or low blood pressure? Is the venous pressure raised? Is arterial perfusion and oxygen saturation adequate? Is there significant oedema? Is the patient anaemic? Or Icteric? Is there an abdominal pain or mass, where is it located and is it tender to palpation? Neurological information will be interesting: Is there any specific sensory or motor disturbance in any area, abnormal gait or unsteadiness? Is there abnormality on ophthalmic examination of the fundus? And so it goes on.

Will a correct diagnosis be achieved or will the patient then be obliged to make a further *delayed* personal visit to the GP to solve what may be a serious acute problem or will he or she be then referred to an A and E Department because such a diagnostic assessment is unsafe. What computer obsessed half wit has persuaded some non-medically trained managers that this will reduce problems of attendance in clinic numbers at the expense of clinical safety? Please come out of your virtual reality bubble into real life. The litigation lawyers must be rubbing their hands! Similarly, the recent recommendation that patients should consult their local pharmacy or other lay practitioners rather than trouble their doctor seems a situation fraught with dangerous possibilities.

(iv) *Staffing Problems*: That Medicine is now obviously regarded as a 'job' is again well illustrated by the recent political statement that finance will be made available for 5000 new doctors and 20,000 new nurses to be magically introduced into the system in the next four to five years. Where are these experienced professionals to come from? If they are to be trained to standards acceptable in this country, it will take at least five to ten years and when qualified the doctors may then not be particularly interested in life as a General Practitioner.

A similar situation will also arise with the Nursing Profession. Nurses take at least three years to be fully trained. How are 20,000 trainee appointments suddenly going to appear or will these nurses be recruited from elsewhere or from countries where standards are lower than those we would expect in the UK? No mention has been made of the linguistic problems that employing more Foreign Nationals will surely ensue.

(v) *The Internal Market*: The other managerial introduction some time ago of the internal market seems to have made little difference to patient care. Patients have not been impressed that their own practitioners have been able to strike a cheap deal for their hospital treatment. Treatment is either good or bad irrespective of the financial basis of its acquisition. How precisely has giving the General Practitioner funds to purchase hospital treatment for their patients achieved any improvement in their care? The bureaucratic consequences of this decision must have been considerable! Surely, it would have been financially more sensible to upgrade some of the facilities in local health centres.

(vi) *Waiting Lists*: The Administrations' alarming suggestion to one group of hospitals some time ago that to clear a two year waiting list of non-urgent conditions within three months no new patients should be treated.

'Sorry you may die of a bleeding peptic ulcer, while someone has their ingrowing toenail treated.' Excellent thinking!

(vii) *Statins and Dementia*: Other splendid dictats have also regularly emerged such as all persons over 50 should be placed on statins, even if not ill. A decision based on questionable evidence. Also that doctors who diagnose patients with dementia should be awarded £55 per person so labelled for whatever clinical reason I cannot conceive. I presume if one achieves 10 diagnoses in a month one is in the running for the £500 Ministry of Health prize!

(viii) *Finally, we have the "home computer diagnostic system"* about to commence that will relieve the A and E Departments and hopefully the General Practitioners from ever having to actually come into physical contact with a human patient. Potential sufferers can now reach for their computers and self-diagnose the cause of their abdominal problems ranging from:

A. Pain

Cholecystitis
Cholelithiasis
Appendicitis
Diverticulosis
Diverticulitis

B. Carcinoma

Stomach
Pancreas
Colon
Rectum
Kidney
Liver
Bladder

C. General Infection

Paratyphoid, Typhoid
Cholera
Dengue Fever
Urinary Tract Infection/Septicaemia
Childhood infections Viz. measles,
    chickenpox and meningitis

D. Vascular

Dissection of the Aorta
Obstruction of — Coeliac Artery
              — Renal Artery
              — Iliac Artery
              — Splenic Artery
              — Carotid Artery

E. Gynaecological

Menorrhagia
Salpingitis
Ectopic Pregnancy
Ovarian Tumours

To mention but a few diagnoses they may come across. With any luck, some may hit the correct target but at least it will give the hypochondriacs a great day out. Having made their diagnosis, what is the patient then supposed to do about it? Presumably, consult and instruct his or her own physician on the treatment that should be delivered. All success to the clinic of Dr Google!

So just few of the Grand Managerial Solutions to the current problems faced by General Practitioners on a daily basis. At least, everything is being recorded by computer to prove how well the managerial element is performing even if the clinical sector appears to be suffering from a significant shortfall in facilities.

One may just finally pose the question 'Why has this situation been allowed to develop with more administrative Staff being employed than Clinicians?' Is it because General Practice has been starved of facilities compared to those given to the Hospital Sector a feature that has been Barn Door obvious for 25 years?!

2. The Practice of Nursing

Much comment has been made about the lack of care and compassion exhibited by some present day nurses. There were obviously problems developing at least thirty years ago when I observed a distinct change in nursing attitudes at Barts.

When I started on the Wards at Barts, they were clearly organised by and under the very direct control of the very competent Ward Sister. It was this lady who ruled and organised the local structure of the whole nursing process. She taught the nurses exactly how a patient should be cared for round the clock and also how a nurse should personally behave towards a patient. Her ward was her empire and the reputation of each ward depended entirely on her efforts and attitude aimed to achieve the high standards expected at St Bartholomew's Hospital. Some wards were notable because of their strict but effective discipline. Some were more relaxed but woe betide any that dropped below the level expected of a London teaching hospital. They were inspected by more Senior Sisters almost daily and also by the Matron who visited all the wards in the hospital regularly once a week. For many these ladies of mature years, the

Ward was their 'life' and not a few of them had been in post for 20 years or more. They were 'the glue' that held the whole hospital together. Incidentally, they also instructed many of the junior doctors — they had seen it and dealt with it all!

Nurses trained in this system permeated to hospitals throughout the country and built very satisfactory systems of nursing worldwide.

Then Hooray… The managerial wand was waved and the whole system was 'improved' by the Salmon Nursing Structure. Seniority was determined by a number starting at the bottom with a nurse in first year training as number 1 and stretching up to the Matron (now Chief Nursing Officer) number 10. To progress in nursing one had to pass through the numbered system with a Ward Sister now being a number 6. A number 7 was a more superior person who was supposed to organise a number of wards and instruct the sisters at number 6.

The whole scheme was based on an industrial pattern devised by Mr Salmon of Joseph Lyons and Co and which was excellent for making Swiss Rolls, Ice-Creams and biscuits but unfortunately now defunct!

These established Ward Sisters were encouraged to climb onto this ascending scale. Guess what! These now number 6s said they did not want to move away from what was for many was their life's work. The last straw was when after a year or so they were bypassed by young ladies or gentlemen on the rise to number 7 who began to dictate to these vastly experienced independent persons and suggest to a Sister of 25 years' service 'I don't think you are running your ward correctly.' The reaction, and it is well recorded, was that over a 3–4-year period nearly 70% of the established Ward sisters at Barts either resigned or retired early leaving the nursing process under the care of less experienced staff. Some of the newly appointed younger persons tried extremely hard to maintain the status quo and also initiate some of the techniques required by newer medical developments but then apparently gave up reportedly due to the attitude of the managerial number 7s and above. I frequently I discussed such problems with these persons on the wards at that period and understood their feelings of being manipulated by persons for whom they had little professional respect.

From this time onwards, as far as I was concerned, the whole process began to deteriorate and patient care began to veer towards the present day system and we all know directly or indirectly what this is now like. Despite these strictures, some nurses ran perfectly acceptable wards but the length of term in office of many number 6s was brief either from progression up the system which incidentally resulted in increased managerial numbers or because of frustration with their lack of autonomy. One or two years in the post was not uncommon and was responsible for much of the lack of continuity that has so sadly emerged. Vastly increasing levels of documentation were required by various managerial systems designed to demonstrate the improved efficiency in the nursing process but which resulted in a burgeoning bureaucracy and less time available for hands on direct patient care. We then had 'degreed' nurses and the bedside functions were devolved to far less trained so-called nursing assistants often coming from other nationalities with very different ethical attitudes to those of this country.

With the European working time directive and other restrictive targets, it does not surprise me that the very personal care and continuity that I knew 30–40 years ago appears to have been almost completely lost with the speed of passage through the system ward nursing staff barely know the name of a patient other than as 'that gall bladder in number 8'. Although many forms have to be filled to ensure that the management process has been completed, much of the 'humanity' has drained away. So "well done the industrialisation of British Nursing." I now await the criticism of the present day Senior Nursing hierarchy who appear to consider what has been achieved a miracle of efficiency and a considerable advance in the status of the nursing profession. The current opinions of the neglected and poorly treated patients might be a little different! Don't worry Dear, your Nurse has a degree but is not quite sure which way the Bed Pan should be applied! He/She will be back in an hour or so when the Computer has been consulted!

3. The Effects on Surgical Practice

I have indicated in much of the narrative the changes that were occurring in the modes of operative procedures in my address at the Royal College of Surgeons in 1993. I suggested that we were not equipping the newly appointed Consultant Staff with the type or length of training that would be necessary to encompass the development of more complex interventional techniques which were becoming dependent upon advanced instrumental systems.

In recent years, it is good to see the increasing number of practical workshops and training programmes that have begun to emerge. There still appear to be some gaps in the system as is revealed by the evidence that some Consultants or Junior staff are carrying out procedures for which they have had insufficient instruction or experience leading to reported clinical disaster.

Surely, this is another situation that would seldom have occurred 30 years ago in the days of the 'Firm' system mentioned above. Here, each trainee passed through a series of graded appointments supervised by Consultant members of one unit who on a day to day basis worked with and intimately knew the capabilities of their juniors and who would have been unlikely to allow them to proceed to full independence until they were considered adequately competent.

Current training programmes still seem inadequate in a number of ways and important in this is the often intermittent and rapid flit of trainees from post to post. These short periods of exposure to practical hands on surgery in the operating theatre are clearly inadequate. The European working time directive is responsible for the diminished time that a trainee can spend on achieving experience with 'hands on' surgical operating. It would appear that this vital period has become reduced to almost half the time that I experienced 30 years ago. I know full well that despite the ten years I spent in surgical training I felt I was only just fully competent at the end of this period. Perhaps I was a slow learner but I cannot conceive how someone can be regarded as a trained surgeon and ready to go completely solo in four to five years. One has just not met and *dealt* with all the difficult situations that will be experienced. There is also the rapid geographical changes of employment that now disrupt family and social life for the trainee.

This lack of a stable continuity in training is certainly an area that needs attention. There seems to be a mild return to the 'Firm' system coupled with the ministerial suggestion that the patient might even benefit by knowing the names of the responsible Consultant and junior staff and by having a notice to that effect over the ward bed. Quite like old times!

It also seems apparent that after a long period of being ignored by various Governments, the advice of the Royal Colleges is being taken seriously again and some of their recommendations acknowledged and accepted. Namely, the gradual repeal of some of the idiocy of the working time directive which has so interfered with the whole of surgical practice. There may be hope that further recommendations will be accepted. It is, however, vitally important that our professional leaders should be supported in their recommendations and independence and do not become unwittingly flattered, massaged and absorbed into the Governmental determined scenario!

In this period of my time in surgical practice, these are just a few of the radical changes I have observed. Many of these decisions I am sure would have appalled those engaged in medical and nursing practice prior to 1948. Some problems may be solved but this will hardly reproduce the same caring attitudes of most practitioners that I knew when I started down this long road and whom I attempted to emulate.

First — A Few Remedial Suggestions From the Past (the 1990s)

In an article in the *British Medical Journal* as long ago as 1994 I suggested that one solution to solving some of these problems might be that if more funding had been made available to the General Practitioner in the nature of providing comprehensive local Health Centres equipped with basic facilities such as simple X-ray and blood analysis facilities, then

(a) the patients would not need to make long journeys,
(b) A and E would not be congested by such patients who had often given up after an impossibly long wait for a routine hospital appointment and
(c) if the old local Cottage Hospital concept was revived, a number of patients requiring only minor interventional day case or one night stay observational facilities or procedures could well be treated by the same very competent General Practitioners entirely LOCALLY and the District General Hospitals and A and E Departments would be relieved of considerable pressure. Some specialisation among a group of practitioners would be helpful without risking the *vital* 'continuity factor' that has now been lost. Also, a number of fully trained nurses living locally might be enticed back to work on a part time basis to fit in with their other commitments. Some facilities of this nature have appeared in limited numbers and appear very successful. But sadly in many areas they have not developed.

Secondly, not all District General Hospitals have the facilities or time for the rapid examination and treatment of patients with more complex or rare conditions which should surely be dealt with in a limited number of specialist institutions arranged on a regional basis such as the Postgraduate Hospitals and Institutes so thoughtfully closed down!

This at last is beginning to happen and is hopefully relieving pressure on the District General Hospitals who are now being forced to close their A and E Services! This seems a fashionable but unpopular solution for local communities with undiagnosed patients then needing to be transported over long distances by stretched ambulance services to mega units. I have no details of the number of patients with minor injuries and conditions which could still be treated in conventional A and E Departments leaving more complex cases to be conveyed directly and treated in comprehensive regional centres. It would also seem logical that these relatively small and active A and E centres should remain functional as is the wish of most local populations.

Most vitally and an immediate necessity is the Urgent Development of an Adequate System of TRIAGE!

A comprehensible and sensible system of Triage should urgently be introduced to separate and refer these various categories of patients to the most appropriate venue at an early stage of their illness decided and originated by an easily accessible *SENIOR AND EXPERIENCED PHYSICIAN* and *NOT* by unqualified telephone operators.

Such arrangements are now grinding into actuality in some areas to relieve a looming situation that was totally obvious 25–30 years ago to many medical and nursing staff. The recent bizarre solutions recorded above are now being presented in the media as sudden and brilliant thinking by guess who? "Another layer of computerised managerial box tickers" boosted by out of touch, gullible politicians who are never backward or anonymous in shouting their new ideas or initiatives in the hope of securing a few more votes.

It was also obvious to many clinicians that almost all these previously suggested facilities were available in embryo and on the ground early on and at quite reasonable cost could have been improved and brought up to date. This could have been achieved more cheaply and without enormous managerial interference with its industrially based concept of the questionable and entirely theoretical advantages of vast centralised organisations. Building larger and larger District General Hospitals does little to ease the local pressure on the General Practitioners. Why did no one look into the medical/nursing suggestion box? It was avoided by the managers and theorists who knew better with their own agendas to pursue and with little regard to the realities of primary medical practice.

Finally, it is worth remarking that the suggestion by management that these problems might be relieved by reordering the training of a doctor or surgeon by methods developed for airline pilots or production line operatives can hardly be compared to the complexity of the human state.

A man or woman's autonomous reactions made up of around three trillion separate cells can have little relation to atmospheric changes over the Atlantic or a Toyota car where the completed machine consists of 1500–4000 parts and rarely exhibits a change in attitude when once assembled. Vide the remarks of Mr Taylor already quoted above.

Again, an example of theoretical Blue Sky Thinking! Why not try speaking to a Dr or a Surgeon!

Chapter 34

The Final Words

The Health Service, a large, worthy and initially an altruistic organisation, has been politically protected by many governments over a 50-year period.

It was obviously necessary at the start to erect an administrative machinery to control the various elements that this enormous concept engendered and the main player at this stage was the medical profession which needed a degree of administrative direction to make the project work. As far as I can ascertain or remember, the bulk of the profession worked ethically and humanely to make it successful. Of course, there were some bad apples but most patients still regarded their doctors with respect at this time for their dedication to their wellbeing.

As the machinery moved into action, it became obvious that this independent and unpredictable part of the organisation needed to be brought to heel. Slowly, slowly this has been achieved but has unfortunately brought about the demise of some of the most important and cherished elements of medical practice.

While I was happily gaining fulfilment in this older system and treating patients on the basis of clinical need, the whole foundation of medical practice was being re-aligned by management and government in to an organisation which for various reasons does not currently provide *all* patients with the standard of care they desire and deserve.

While enlightened control is necessary, it has become financially difficult to dispense a satisfactory package of medical care in such an ambitious but underfunded organisation to an expanding and ageing population. In previous chapters, I have tried to identify just a few of the reasons for the dissatisfactions that have emerged and are reported by patients.

I am convinced and have tried to highlight that one of the most significant causes of such unhappiness is the corruption of the hallowed 'one-to-one' relationship that always needs to be established between patient and doctor. The patient when unwell seeks the advice of a trusted and familiar professional individual with whom he or she has adequate time to discuss their problems, be listened to and if appropriate accept the recommended pathway towards normal health. All else is entirely peripheral to this 'key' relationship with the highly valued and sought 'humanity factor' at its centre. Nursing and technical assistance is obviously necessary but is ancillary to this primacy of the physician.

Currently, the interposition of a third party such as government or management by dictat significantly disturbs this relationship at the considerable risk of patient dissatisfaction should this intervention not be sensible or sympathetic and continuity of care begins to fragment.

It is here that government for political reasons or management for inherent dislike of this very personal relationship has I believe deliberately sidelined the advisory nature of the professions and a patient must now be brought to realise that a physician has become a full time civil servant and any thoughts of independent action must be curtailed.

For example, the Government and its medical and non-medically trained advisors sporadically release quite peculiar statements of intent such as those noted in the previous chapter. Also, non-medically trained management has recently started to issue bullying and quite unbelievable local directives which engender a degree of anger and unhappiness rather than co-operation in their prime professional staff at the work face. Threats of dismissal for highlighting deficiencies in the service are not helpful. It is a wonderful and blinkered organisation that alienates an important and vital proportion of its workforce for telling the truth. It now appears that newly appointed staff are to be instructed on how to complain correctly! Presumably, *they* can then be blamed for *not* having complained correctly when things go wrong.

To those who have not noticed, the bulk of the medical profession is still more interested in treating patients consistently and humanely and does not take kindly to the attitudes currently exhibited by the managerial enthusiasts with their need to confine medical practice into a vast computer format with timetables, targets and numerical lists of requirements and outcomes so redolent of US management speak. They might care to remember the statement of Professor Albert Einstein. 'Not everything that can be counted counts and not everything that counts can be counted' could be well applied to the practice of medicine where 'the patient counts' above all else.

Such practices have unintentional consequences. Among these being the early retirement of a number of surgeons and physicians and their retreat into private practice in order to return to the 'old-fashioned' practice of Medicine with 'treatment by clinical need' and not managerial and monetary convenience. There is also the quiet haemorrhage of young British trained Doctors to appointments abroad where it is still possible to practice Medicine as a Profession and not a Job.

It would appear that management has now almost completed the Establishment of a 'Post Office Counter' type of Medicine staffed by younger members of the professions some of whom appear happy with a '9–5 no weekend' style of limited responsibility as a fully satisfying 'job' and are unfamiliar with an independent 24/7 type of professional ethos of which they have had little or no experience. The new attempt to re-introduce a seven day working system is now causing considerable upheaval with junior medical staff who are not prepared to provide this cover except for a financial consideration whereas in the days of medicine as a profession such care would have been provided as a norm. Another bull's eye for management and government.

It is also of interest to observe how the General Medical Council has subtly come under Government control by adding increasing restrictions and regulation to the independent activity of the medical profession whilst projecting its myth of being an 'Independent Organisational Charity' and interested purely in the revalidation of medical ability but quietly at the same time moulding the physician into the servant of the desired system.

Another systemic consequence of this new regime is that continuity of care and loss of kindness is becoming apparent within hospitals where patients are being moved from appointment to appointment, department to department and from ward to ward for managerial expediency and with insufficient time or opportunity to discuss the investigation or treatment of their condition with a doctor. A situation that is often complicated by deficiencies in the linguistic capability of the newer medical and nursing staff. Practices such as old persons being discharged for expediency to empty unattended accommodation in the middle of the night would have been unbelievable to the medical and nursing staff of forty years ago! Repeatedly cancelled over run of rearranged operation lists by non-medical administrative staff adhering to managerial protocol are ludicrously common and psychologically deeply disturbing for the patient. The most heinous crime when I was working was to cancel a patient's booked operation. Lists were compiled with clinical knowledge and continued until all had been treated. A fact recognised by staff from Consultant to theatre porters with no constriction on time spent. Such recent managerial manipulations have obviously contributed to the huge well of dissatisfaction being experienced by both patients and staff.

Despite the efforts of many different grades of medical and nursing staff who are still providing a superb service in trying to help ill people, other employees are undermining vital parts of the system and rapidly degrading its public reputation with poor performance and lack of professional integrity.

There are certainly staff shortages and underfunding in many areas but injecting further money into the system will not cure these ills which are fundamental examples of human failure by non-medically trained personnel. Patients are not packets of Cornflakes to be moved uncaringly from shelf to shelf in a supermarket for market expediency.

As retirement came upon me, I was thankfully able to continue to practice in private, the type of medicine I had been taught many years ago.

Consultations could be made when desired, each patient having one's full attention for however long it was necessary. Complete examination was possible and the appropriate investigations could be requested without restriction with an answer available within 24 hours instead of 24 days. Any interventional therapy could be carried out under optimum circumstances for both patient and doctor at a mutual time of choice usually within two to three days. Highly qualified consultants in other disciplines could easily be brought into consultation to advise and manage specific problems such as postoperative intensive care or other non-related but important medical conditions.

Obviously, all this can only be achieved at financial cost but nevertheless many elderly patients still remember and desire this 'old type of attention' to be available in the public sector. The Government should surely come clean and clearly state that such a service is just not achievable with the amount of funding and diminishing personal integrity now available and required by such a complex system of Health and Social Security. This should be made known more publically as in the Prime Minister's frequently used phrase 'in a clear and transparent manner' and that patients will have to lower their expectations and learn to tolerate the system that has been developed for them.

It is still a grand but not a unique scheme and one which aspires to be the epitome of health engineering although other countries appear to have achieved much more efficient and 'patient satisfactory' arrangements .This is particularly noticeable in other European States such as Germany, Holland and France. The National Health System will obviously be protected by whatever Government is in power but in its present format it is always destined to be financially constrained. Far better and sensible *intelligent* management would be the most likely and rapidly efficient way of improving the system within the financial limitations available and some of the many recent lamentable managerial failures especially by highly paid individuals of questionable intelligence should be corrected and eliminated. Surely the time has come when 'the Management needs to be 'Disciplined' not the Consultant staff! Vide my King Edward VII course of 1968.'

Looking back over all this jumble of one person's experiences what is outstanding.

To me, the principal fact was that despite the occasional unevenness of the road I thoroughly enjoyed my professional life as a doctor and a surgeon. Meeting and getting to know such a variety of many pleasant and interesting persons was always an enormous satisfaction. The technicality of surgery was a prime stimulus and I never felt I was in any way performing in a 'life saving' scenario as is frequently portrayed in the media. Nor did I feel the administrative constraints that many of my younger successors are now experiencing.

As I Travelled Along, Three Salient Areas of Activity Became Apparent

In My Early Years, the Experience of Open Surgery

Within the accepted practices of the time, I not infrequently saw some surgery which was unnecessarily rough and damaging and was the reason that I looked for other means of alleviating this iatrogenic crudity having seen what could be achieved by the precision of neurosurgery.

I think in the early days of our efforts in ischaemic open renal surgery we were able to considerably improve on the methods currently available at that time.

The Era of Endoscopic Expansion in Surgery and Minimally Invasiveness

It was here that I really experienced a period of excitement while enabling the mechanisms of endoscopic intrarenal surgery, meeting other surgeons of like mind in various specialities and which lead me to the coining of the name 'MINIMALLY INVASIVE SURGERY' as a consequence of the observed lack of morbidity and rapid return to normal health that this more careful type of surgery engendered.

The Era of Robotic Surgery

Having been considerably involved in the development of one of the first types of mechanical approach to improving the accuracy of surgery with the computer based Probot I found that this was the most enlightening period of my surgical life. The potential of this approach is so vast and the introduction of Surgeon Assisted Robotic devices such as the da Vinci instrument imported from the USA has been another critical step forward in interventional medicine. At last, abdominal surgery can be effected without the need to pass large and possibly infected, although gloved, hands, inside a patient's abdomen and thereby achieve a much more accurate endoscopic intervention which is heralding the demise of the crudities of many long established procedures. I hope our efforts over these years may have had some small impact in reducing unnecessary surgical injury to our ever trusting patients.

In 60 years' time, children will be told 'As late as the 2030s and 40s doctors called surgeons were putting their hands inside people's tummies to do operations' How gross! Unbelievable! How quickly this later phase will develop is difficult to predict. If it is to prosper in the UK as of old, physicians should be the principal guide to these processes aided by a far more enlightened attitude of management. One that listens and is supportive rather than being more prescriptive and interested in its own complexities than that of the patients well-being.

From these random observations, I might venture a few predictions. Firstly no matter what eventuates, interventional medicine or surgery will become more mechanistic, more accurate and less traumatic but unfortunately more expensive. The early days of the application of robotic instrumentation have demonstrated that 'stand-alone' robots if suitably programmed can perform an accurate operation without manual input. I can visualise similar procedures being performed in the future with the robot guided by more sophisticated computer diagnostic imaging. The field is open for exploration!

In the medical area, it is obvious that the accelerating impact of genetic analysis upon therapy in general will be immense as more and more of our somatic make-up is being revealed almost daily. The application of various modalities of genetic engineering will ultimately result in significant modifications of cellular behaviour particularly in cancer cell control. Many of the current procedures involving the surgical extirpation of malignant material will be rendered unnecessary with the preservation of the related organ systems and will produce a considerable modification in the conventional surgical repertoire. Such new therapy will inevitably be expensive and how it can be translated into day to day practice will be one of the most challenging problems to face in the next three to four decades? It is all very well to set up a number of centres around the country to provide genomic analysis of patients' problems. But how can the emergent results of such information be translated into therapy without considerable financial enhancement in an environment that seems unable to reliably carry out simple X-rays or scans within a reasonable time span. Has this been thought through? The impact of the need for genetic therapeutic mechanisms will obviously add another immense dimension to the work of the hospitals and pharmaceutical industries, the costs of which will surely be considerable. How will the NHS contain this potentially enormous expense? If patients are to benefit from such advances, I fear many of these costs will have to be borne personally which again will raise considerable political and philosophical problems.

The majority of interventional medicine will still be concerned with more mundane problems but I am sure these will be treated by better planned and less traumatic means as long as the implementation of such emerging techniques is left in the hands of the consultant medical staff. Surgery as a career will still have tremendous and exciting possibilities so long as its evolution will be guided and determined by experienced clinicians who are not confined by a myriad of protocols. It would be of considerable help if the Politicians would back off and allow persons who know the actuality of the situation to guide the projects of surgical and medical advance rather than listening to the blandishments of self-interested lay parties with various agendas to pursue.

More and more decisions on the development of healthcare will, I am sure, be verging on the preventative and physiological rather than the purely clinical treatment of established disease and patients must continue to be educated and be more personally responsible for the care of their bodies by sensible lifestyle modifications. Patients should in general be fit when they die of old age!

Finally, many of my experiences in a surgical life have been exciting and uplifting and the time and freedom to innovate was always a great stimulus and must hopefully be preserved. Now over recent years due to constraints of time and finance this freedom appears to be limited. In the UK, we now pick up emerging techniques second hand from other countries such as Germany, Japan, India, China and the USA vide the imported da Vinci robot assist mechanisms or the specifically designed medications based on a patients independent genomic analysis. This latter being extremely expensive to introduce from another country and to implement in the UK.

Prime innovation now stems from abroad. This is worrying but I do not think it is lack of local talent but is possibly the result of the systemic restrictions that our young surgeons and physicians are increasingly experiencing. A recent review of the scientific programme of the International Society for Medical Innovation and Technology in 2015 showed that not one paper or report emanated from the UK when twenty years ago at least one quarter of about one hundred contributions came from Great Britain. Is this a reflection of some active diversion away from time devoted to innovation? It might be worth enquiring from the politicians and managers why this should be so?

On the positive side, towards the end of my practice two unexpected events occurred. I mentioned many pages ago that I had undertaken a number of my undergraduate examinations in the Society of Apothecaries Hall, Blackfriars, London each time wondering if I would be successful and whether I would ever become a

Doctor. I was therefore totally surprised to be invited as Guest of Honour to a Dinner in the same Hall many years later and was presented with a very flattering citation and the Galen Gold Medal of the Society, their most prestigious award for my services to surgery over 40 odd years.

The Royal College of Surgeons of England subsequently bestowed the Cheselden Medal for my exploits in surgery with similar kind remarks so perhaps in the eyes of some of my colleagues I got a few things right! Occasionally, people hear what one has been trying to say even if it is sometimes distasteful.

In 2012, the European Society of Urology bestowed on me their 'Innovators in Urology' award, another kind Citation and a beautiful bronze facsimile of the whole Urinary Tract. So not just recognition in the UK!

Concomitantly over the last fifty years there has been a gradual dismantling of Medicine as an independent profession.

Here in the United Kingdom, the majority of Physicians have become direct employees of the State. Control until recently has been benign and generally well tolerated. Now the Government has revealed its controlling hand and unilaterally directed the junior Medical staff to do its bidding. How long will it be before a similar control will be extended to the Senior staff?

It has taken a long time for the Physicians to appreciate that the days of professional independence have ended and that they, as paid employees, are subject to the rough and tumble of economic reality.

I fear that the days of the kind old GP who called twice a day to treat my Scarlet Fever are well and truly past.

A shadow of independent medical practice may still persist in the private sector but for how long I would not like to predict.

John Wickham
2016

Appendix 1

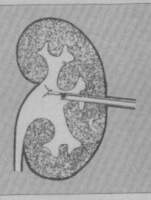

Practical Course Percutaneous Renal Surgery and Radiology

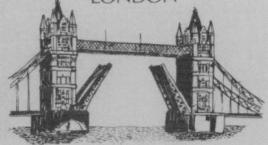

INSTITUTE OF UROLOGY
LONDON

20-22 Sept 1983

Appendix 2

THE SOCIETY OF
MINIMALLY INVASIVE SURGERY

INAUGURAL MEETING

at

THE ROYAL INSTITUTION

LONDON

11–12 DECEMBER 1989

ORGANISERS

J E A WICKHAM   J M FITZPATRICK

THE SOCIETY OF MINIMALLY INVASIVE SURGERY INAUGURAL MEETING AT THE ROYAL INSTITUTION LONDON 11–12 DECEMBER 1989 ORGANISERS

J E A WICKHAM   J M FITZPATRICK

MONDAY — 11 DECEMBER 1989

MORNING SESSION

Chairman: Mr J E A Wickham

Introduction

10.00–10.15 **The Concept**	J E A Wickham, UK
10.15–10.45 **Gastroenterology**	Professor G Buess, Germany
	Professor F Dubois, France
10.45–11.15 **Urology**	Professor F Eisenburger, Germany
	Professor D P Griffiths, USA
11.30–12.00 **Gynaecology**	Professor K Semm, Germany
	Dr H Reich, USA
12.00–12.30 **Orthopaedics**	Mr D Dandy, UK

AFTERNOON SESSION

Chairman: *Professor J M Fitzpatrick*

2.00–2.30 **ENT**	Professor H Stammburger, Austria
	Professor W Steiner, Germany
2.30–3.00 **Neurosurgery**	Mr D Thomas, UK
3.00–3.30 **Cardiovascular**	Professor D J Allison, UK

3.30–4.00 **General Surgery**   Professor R Wittmoser, Germany
Dr E J Reddick, USA
4.30–5.30 **General Open Discussion**

EVENING

INAUGURAL SOCIETY DINNER

at the
BARBER SURGEONS HALL
MONKWELL SQUARE CITY OF LONDON

TUESDAY — 12 DECEMBER 1989

DISCUSSION DAY

9.00–9.30   **Minimal Invasive Surgery and the Integration of the Specialities**
Mr J E A Wickham, UK
Professor J M Fitzpatrick, Ireland

9.30–10.00   **Training Programmes in Minimal Invasive Surgery**
Professor K Semm, Germany Dr A Smith, USA

10.00–10.30   **Minimal Invasive Surgery and the Change from General to Local Anaesthesia**
Professor J C Whitwam, UK

10.30–11.00   **The Change from Inpatient to Outpatient Surgery**
Professor J W Segura, USA Mr R Miller, UK

11.30–12.00   **Imaging Technology — Future Developments**
Professor D J Allison, UK

2.00–2.30   **Integration of the Clinicians and Manufacturers**
Mr R Vickers, UK

2.30–4.00   **The Manufacturer's Point of View**

Speakers Dr P Hooper (Roche Products Limited)
Dr H Wurster (Richard Wolf)
Mr S Greengrass (Olympus Limited)
Mr R Koller (Storz)
Mr J Abele (Radiologic)
Mr A C Hicks (William Cook Ltd)
Mr H Furamoto (Candela Corp)
Dr H J Mager (Dornier)

4.30–5.30 **The Future of the Society**
Mr J E A Wickham, UK
Professor J M Fitzpatrick, Ireland

When, where, format, journal, a foundation? Please think about these question.

DELEGATES AND COUNTRIES OF ORIGIN

Abele J	USA	Manegola BC	Germany
Adwers J	USA	Marberger M	Austria
Allison DJ	UK	Mardis HK	USA
Bagley D	USA	McColl I	UK
Bonnet L	Germany	Miller R	UK
Bowen S	UK	Molgaard-Nielsen A	UK
Buess G	Germany	Nathanson K	UK
Chiverton S	UK	Perissat J	France
Clayman R	USA	Pittas M	UK
Coptcoat M	UK	Popp LW	Germany
Cumberland DC	UK	Prophet MJ	UK
Dandy D	UK	Quint R	USA
Dubois P	France	Rassweiler J	Germany
Eisenberger P	Germany	Reddick E	USA
Ell Ch	Germany	Reich H	USA

Fitzpatrick JM	Ireland	Rimmer PG	UK
Freidich JP	France	Russell C	UK
Fuchs G	USA	Segura J	USA
Furamoto H	USA	Semm K	Germany
Gautier JR	France	Simon P	Switzerland
Greengrass S	UK	Smith A	USA
Griffith D	USA	Stammberger H	Austria
Hatfield AR	UK	Starr G	UK
Hauer G	Germany	Steiner W	Germany
Hicks AH	UK	Tan H	Australia
Holdoway ATJ	UK	Thomas D	UK
Holmes F	UK	Thomson K	Australia
Hooper P	UK	Treat MR	USA
Ikeuchi H	Japan	Vallencien G	France
Jipp P	Germany	Van den Branden E	UK
Kasinkas M	USA	Vickers R	UK
Kasper B	Switzerland	Watson G	UK
Keckstein J	Germany	Webb D	Australia
Kellett M	UK	Weist FM	Germany
Kirkham J	UK	White BG	UK
Koller R	Germany	Whitfield H	UK
Korth Knut	Germany	Whitwam JG	UK
Lewis R	UK	Wickham JEA	UK
Lucas B	USA	Williams C	UK
MacKay Ian	UK	Wittmoser R	Germany
Mager HJ	Germany	Wurster H	Germany
Magos A	UK	Yoshida O	Japan

Appendix 3

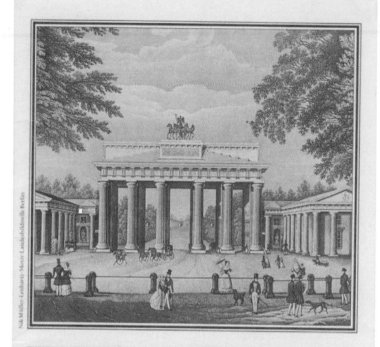

THE SOCIETY
FOR MINIMALLY INVASIVE THERAPY
SMIT
SIXTH INTERNATIONAL MEETING 1994
2–4 OCTOBER, 1994
HOTEL INTER*CONTINENTAL BERLIN

With friendly support of the Senator for Economics & Technology in Berlin within the scope of MEDTECH '94 and the "Society for Promotion of Research, Technology, Presentation and Training in Medicine and Techniques"

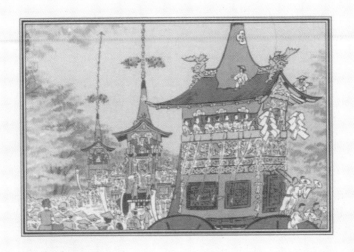

THE SOCIETY
FOR MINIMALLY INVASIVE THERAPY
SMIT
9TH ANNUAL INTERNATIONAL MEETING
JULY 14 - 16, 1997
Kyoto International Conference Hall, Kyoto, Japan

Second Circular
Call for Papers and Registration